Encyclopedia of Medical Elementology

S.B. Vohora

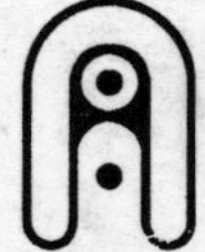

NEW AGE INTERNATIONAL (P) LIMITED, PUBLISHERS
(formerly Wiley Eastern Limited)
New Delhi • Bangalore • Chennai • Guwahati • Hyderabad
• Jalandar •Kolkata • Lucknow • Mumbai • Ranchi
Visit us at **www.newagepublishers.com**

Published by New Age International (P) Ltd., Publishers
First Edition: 2007

ISBN : 81-224-1992-5

Rs. 395.00

C-06-09-1044

Printed in India at Chaman Offset, Delhi.
Typeset at Classic Computers, Delhi.

PUBLISHING FOR ONE WORLD

NEW AGE INTERNATIONAL (P) LIMITED, PUBLISHERS
(formerly Wiley Eastern Limited)
4835/24, Ansari Road, Daryaganj, New Delhi - 110002
Visit us at **www.newagepublishers.com**

Dedicated to

Late Hakeem Abdul Hameed

who conceived the concept of
Medical Elementology

आचार्य एन. के. गांगुली
महानिदेशक
Prof. N.K. Ganguly
MD. D.Sc. (hc) FRC Path. (London), FAMS,
FNA, FASc, FNASc
FTWAS (Italy), FIACS (Canada), FIMSA
Director General

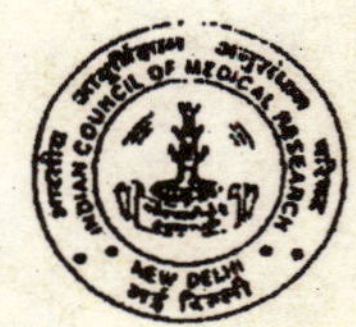

भारतीय आयुर्विज्ञान अनुसंधान परिषद
वी. रामलिंगस्वामी भवन, अंसारी नगर,
पोस्ट बॉक्स 4911, नई दिल्ली-110029,
Indian Council of Medical Research
V. Ramalingaswami Bhawan, Ansari Nagar
Post Box 4911, New Delhi - 110029

FOREWORD

I am happy to know that Prof. S.B.Vohora, former Head, Department of Medical Elementology and Toxicology, Hamdard University, New Delhi has come out with an Encyclopedia of Medical Elementology.

The Five-Element Theory is an important part of oriental medicine and Eastern philosophy in general. Earth, Water, Air, Fire and Space are the five elements in oriental medicine, which refer to five categories in the natural world. This theory holds that all phenomena in the world correspond to these elements, and are in state of constant motion and change. We now know that the number of elements is 106+. Majority of them is present in the human body. It is the complex balance of appropriate amounts of these elements, which is vital for the health of a human being.

I congratulate Prof. Vohora for bringing forth such an exhaustive volume on the distribution of various elements in the ecosystem, their safe levels in drinking water, the food sources from which individual elements can be obtained and the role of the various elements in health and disease.

(N.K. Ganguly)

Director General

Tele : 26588204 (Off); PABX: 26589334, 26589335, 26589336, 26588707, Ext : 264 Res : 26493145, 26493045 Fax: 91-11-26588662, 26589492, 26589647, 26589258, E-mail-icmrhqds@sansad.nic.in. ganguly@icmr.delhi.nic.in

PREFACE

Medical Elementology is envisaged as a new discipline in science wherein constituent elements of the human body form the basis of etiology, pathogenesis, diagnosis and therapy of diseases. It is a unique synthesis of ancient philosophical concepts and modern sciences. Two ancient concepts: (*i*) Human body is a microcosm which reflects Nature as macrocosm, and (*ii*) Organized state of elements represents health and their imbalance causes diseases, were scrutinized in the light of present-day knowledge and global dialogue (four international conferences). Probably the key to all human ailments is hidden within the body necessitating a better understanding and utilization of our own resources. This volume embodies: (*a*) Description of the concept and its development, (*b*) Short monographs on 92 naturally-occurring elements. The coverage includes Category, Distribution in ecosystems, Role, Deficiency, Metabolism, Systemic effects, Intake, Requirements, Medicinal uses, Toxicity, and Guideline values, (*c*) Diseases associated with deficiency and over-exposure of elements, and (*d*) Clinical applications (diagnostic and therapeutic uses or potential). Global interest in the role of elements in human health and disease indicates that Medical Elementology has immense potential for development. It is hoped that the book will stimulate many more workers in this field of research for human benefit.

Chapter 1: Medical Elementology has been reproduced from my earlier work: *New Horizons of Health Aspects of Elements* published by Hamdard University, New Delhi in 1990. Extensive citations for data on elemental content in the ecosystems, guideline values, intake and requirements and some parts of the text have been made from *Metals and Their Compounds in the Environment* (Ed., E. Merian) published by VCH, Weinheim in 1991. Similar citations were made for some metals from our earlier publication: *Heavy Metals and Environment* by M. Athar and S.B. Vohora published by Wiley Eastern/New Age International, New Delhi in 1995. Permissions granted, on behalf of the publishers, by Mr. Siraj Hussain, Vice Chancellor, Hamdard University, New Delhi, India, Ms Bettina Loycke, Copyright and Licensing Manager, Wiley-VCH Verlag GmbH & Co, KG, Weinheim, Germany and Mr. Saumya Gupta, Managing Director, New Age International Publishers New Delhi, India are gratefully acknowledged. My students deserve special appreciation for contributing to this volume from their M. Pharm. (Pharmacology) and Ph. D. (Toxicology) theses: M/s Kulbushan Ganotra (1992), Ayesha Nadeem (1999), Sonia Bajaj (1999), Rumana Siddiqui (2000), Gyan Vikash Mishra (2000) and Zahoor Ahmad Shah (2001). Thanks are due to Mr. Mueed Ahmad and Ms. Neda Ashraf for excellent secretarial assistance.

New Delhi,

September 2006

S.B. Vohora

New Delhi — S.B. Vohora

September 200[illegible]

CONTENTS

1

MEDICAL ELEMENTOLOGY

The two most prevalent systems of medicine in India are Ayurveda (*Ayu*: Life, *Veda*: Science) or the Science of life and Unani-Tibb or the Greco-Arab system of medicine. Over the centuries of practice, there has been considerable intermingling of the two systems of medicine in India, each adopting some concepts and drugs from the other. A '*holistic*' approach involving a perfect balance or equilibrium of elements, temperaments and humours is discernible in the concepts of both Ayurveda and Unani-Tibb.

ARKAN (elements), AKHLAT (humours) and MIZAJ (temperaments) constitute the basis of Unani-Tibb. According to Greco-Arab system of medicine, there are four elements; ATISH (fire), AAB (water), BAD (air) and KHAK (earth).

Ayurveda describes five elements, the fifth being AKASH (space). The concept of elements has recently been studied in details (in the light of modern chemistry, nutrition, physiology and medicine) at the Institute of History of Medicine and Medical Research, New Delhi. The questions that we have been asking ourselves are:

- What is life?
- What is the relation of Man and his Environment?
- Is human body a Microcosm or a Mini-universe?
- Are these questions important for philosophers only and irrelevant for health scientists?

A unique conference : First International Conference on Elements in Health and Disease held in 1983 at New Delhi[12] showed that it is not so. On the contrary, joint deliberations by about 100 scientists of various disciplines from 18 countries of the world, probably laid the foundation for a new discipline in science: Medical Elementology. Nobel laureate Prof. M.H.F. Wilkins from U.K., speaking on this occasion, stressed the need for a 'holistic' approach to the problem of human suffering and rightly pointed out that "time has come for philosophy to say interesting things to science".

Ancient Theories

'AHAM BRAHMASMI' is a Sanskrit quotation from ancient Hindu scriptures which means, "I am the Universe". Philosophers of the Greco-Arab medicine also believe: "Man as microcosm reflects nature as macrocosm". Human body has been described as a microcosm or a mini-universe. Late Hakeem Abdul Hameed, Chancellor, Hamdard University, New Delhi and an exponent of Greco-Arab (Unani) system of medicine posed many stimulating and thought-provoking questions in this context. He argued that if human body is really a microcosm, it should be a combination or manifestation of all material processes or forces and should possess all the elements that are present in nature.[193]

We know now, the number of elements is not four or five (earth, water, air, fire and space), as preached in Unani and Ayurvedic philosophies, but there are 106+ elements in the Periodic Table. So, if the ancient theories stand the test of time and scientific scrutiny, all of these elements must be present in the human body.

Investigation

A survey of world literature was, therefore, conducted to unearth what is known on the subject and analyse the available data for a critical appraisal of the problem. The study[193,196] revealed that 81 elements have been reported to be present in the human body to date (Figure 1).

This means that only 25 elements have not been detected in the human body so far. These include 14 artificial or man-made elements; the number of naturally-occurring elements being 92. The remaining 11 include 5 inert gases (Ar, He, Kr, Ne, Xe). The absence of these elements in the human body can be attributed to the fact that they are unable to react with other compounds because of their inert nature. This leaves out only 6 elements (Actinium, Astatine, Francium, Proctactinium,

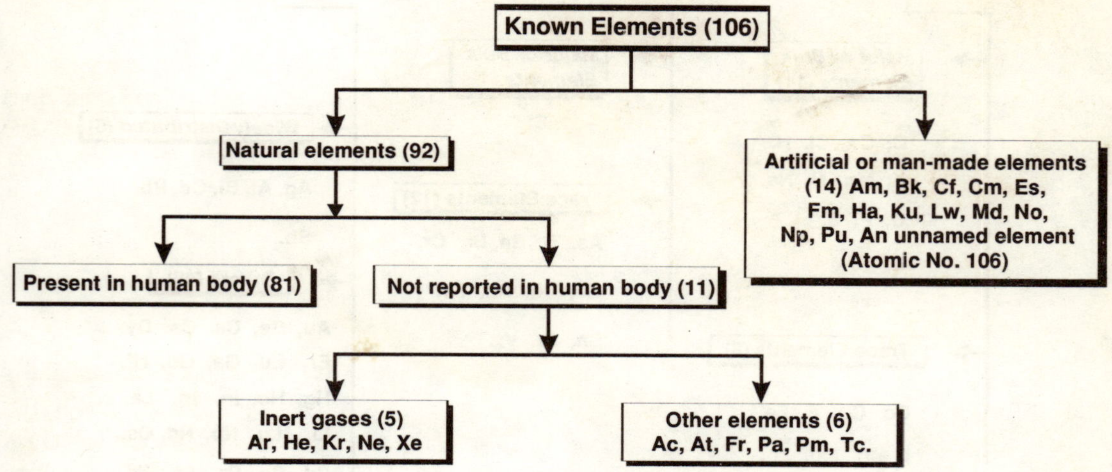

Fig .1 : Elements in the Human Body

Promethium, Technitium) which have not been reported in the human body. We do not know whether human tissues and body fluids were analysed for these elements or studies were made to establish their presence or absence. As the number of elements found in the human body has been steadily increasing, it will not be proper to classify any element as being absent in the human system. The number has shot up from a mere 18 about 60 years ago to 81 today. Do these facts nearly prove that human body is a microcosm? Prof. Nielsen of the Human Nutrition Research Laboratory, North Dakota (USA) in a personal communication[132] to us remarked: "I tend not to believe that man is a microcosm or a combination or manifestation of all materials and other forces. For example, it is likely that the human body contains all elements (present analytical technology prevents this from being a definite statement). However, the majority of these elements are probably there as contaminants from the environment, not as essential components of man". This led us to a study of biological classification of elements (Figure 2).

The objection is very valid since no known functions have, so far, been attributed to as many as 49 elements. But this should be viewed in the light of the following facts:

1. Biological classification of elements is fluid. Many elements (*e.g.*, As, Ba, B, Br, Cr, Ni, Si, Sn, V, etc.), which were hitherto considered non-essential or accumulative (or in the words of Porf. Nielsen, contaminants), have in recent years been shifted to the category of possibly essential elements. As late as in 1971, it was stated that some metals are relatively abundant in Earth's crust but are not found *in vivo e.g.*, Cr and Ni because they are so strongly held in minerals that they are unable to enter plants and then our bodies[212], but

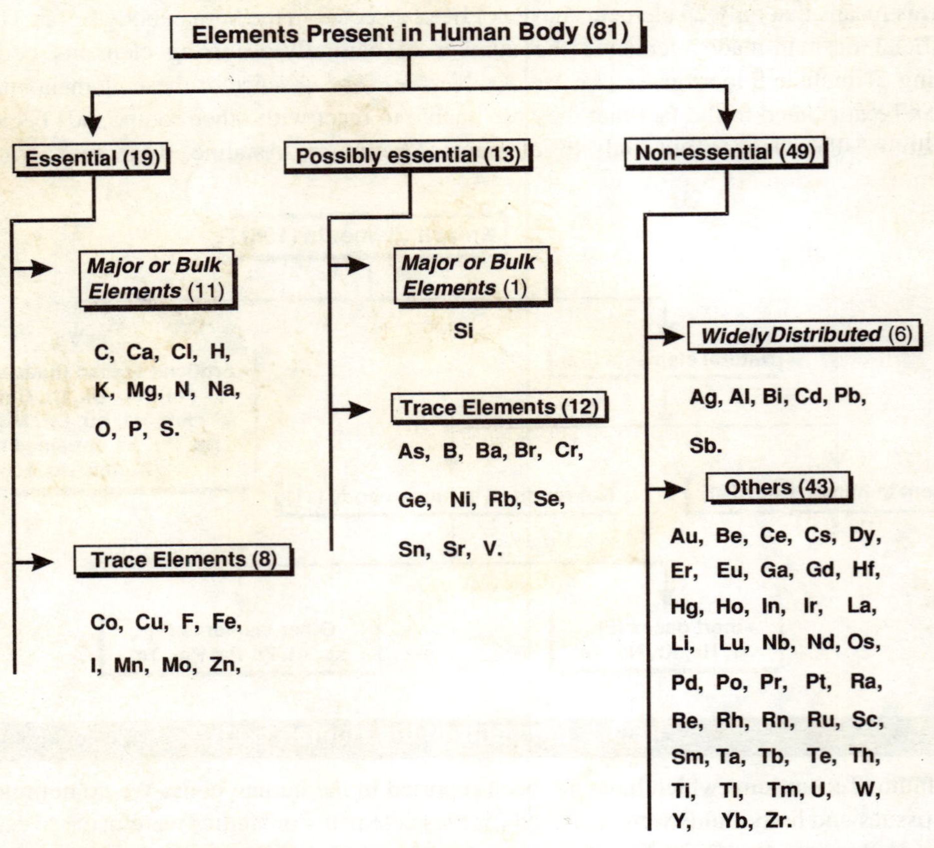

Fig. 2 : Biological Classification of Elements.

later not only their presence was reported, they were even shown to have some essential functions. There is no reason to believe that essential functions will not be discovered for many more elements with the advancement of knowledge.

2. A study was carried out to find out the extent of distribution of 81 elements in 55 human tissues and body fluids. This helped in identification of top 27 elements with wide distribution (in 40 and above body tissues/fluids). The list includes 15 essential (C, H, N, O, Na, K, Ca, Mn, Mg, Cu, Zn, Fe, F, Cl, Co) and 6 possibly essential elements (Ba, Sr, Br, Cr, Sn, Ni). Six elements in this list (Al, Pb, Cd, Ag, Bi, Sb) are, so far, considered non-essential or accumulative elements. Is their presence and such wide distribution in the body (in more than 40 tissues/body fluids) without any purpose or function? We do not know the answer but it is very unlikely because everything in Nature must have a purpose or function to be unveiled with the advancement of knowledge. The present day "contaminants from environment" may then be viewed as "essential components of life". Let us revert to the question: Is human body a microcosm?" I would say that evidence is fast growing in favour of an affirmative answer.

Medical Application

It may be argued even if human body is a microcosm, so what? What are its potential applications? Schroeder[158] stated that many, if not all elements could probably be found in traces in the human tissues if sufficiently sensitive techniques were developed. It would, however, strain human imagination to believe that at such concentrations they could possibly cause adverse or beneficial effects on health. For example, only 5 atoms of Cobalt are present for every billion atoms in the body (Table 1).

Table 1. **Data on Some Elements Present in the Human Body**[14]

Elements	Number of atoms present for every billion atoms in the body
	Million
Hydrogen	630.0
Oxygen	255.0
Carbon	94.5
Nitrogen	13.5
Calcium	3.1
Phosphorus	2.2
	Hundred-Thousand
Potassium	5.7
Sulfur	4.9
Sodium	4.1
Chlorine	2.6
Magnesium	1.3
	Hundred
Manganese	1.7
Copper	1.7
Fluorine	1.2
	Unit
Iodine	20
Molybdenum	10
Cobalt	5

Is it not strange that the body can do with so little and yet is not able to get along with none at all? From five atoms per billion to zero atoms per billion seems such a small step? Not really when we look at the mathematical explanation given by Asimov[14] (Table 2).

Table 2. Cobalt in Human Body

■ Number of atoms present for every billion atoms of the body	:	5
■ Total number of atoms present in each cell	:	9×10^{13}
■ Total number of cells present in the body	:	2.5×10^{13}
■ Cobalt atoms present in each cell	:	4.5×10^{5}
■ Cobalt atoms present in the whole body	:	11.25×10^{18}

It will be seen that 5 Co atoms per billion atoms is equivalent to 450 thousand atoms present in each cell and 11.25 million trillion atoms of Co in the whole body. Hence the difference between 5 and 0 atoms per billion atoms may not seem much, but certainly there is a vast difference between a cell having a few hundred thousand atoms and its having none at all. Target cells (*e.g.*, liver cells in case of Co) may have upto 1-2 million atoms per cell. Iyenger[91] observed, "essentially man is a complex chemical system which reacts to changes in the input of its components which upset its equilibrium, and normality of functioning. Paradoxically, imbalances of trace element nutrition are not characterized by easily recognizable symptoms and marginal deficiencies or excesses which occur relatively frequently, often escape recognition requiring rather sophisticated procedures for indentification".

An Urdu couplet by Chakbast very aptly describes the applied part of the Unani concept. It says:

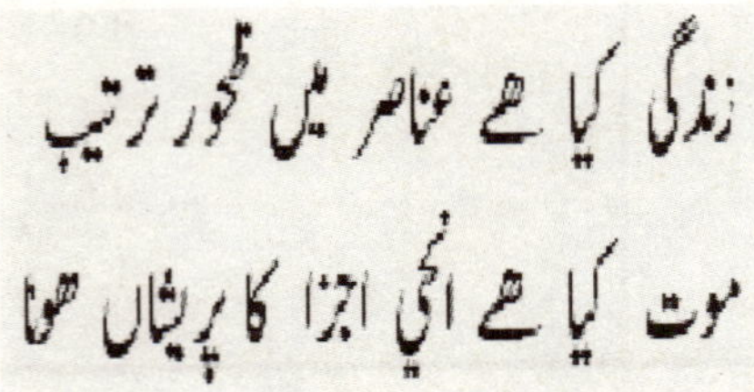

जिन्दगी क्या है, अनासिर में ज़हूरे तरतीब
मौत क्या है, इन्ही अज्ज़ा का परेशां होना

What is life?

– an organized state of elements.

What is death?

– a state of disorder of these components.

Here we interpret 'Life' as 'Health'. When total disorder is 'Death', lesser disorder should mean 'Disease', restoration of the deficient elements (s) or imbalance should be a logical approach to the treatment of disease. Probably the key to all human ailments lies within the body.

A scientific investigation[194] revealed that at least 235 diseases/functions of the human body are affected by its 81 component elements. The effects are brought about by their deficiency, excess or medicinal use. Though only 32/81 elements are considered essential or possibly essential, there are indicators that many more elements affect human health and disease states.

The fields of body composition studies and trace element research are relatively new. With the exception of Fe and I, deficiency states were not recognized for other elements, prior to 1960s. The literature on these subjects is growing rapidly.[36,78,210,211,217] Deliberations at the WHO/IHMMR sponsored First International Conference on Elements in Health and Disease, New Delhi (1983) followed by the formation of International Union of Elementologists (1983) and organization of three subsequent conferences in the series at Karachi (1987), Turkey (1989) and New Delhi (1993) has strengthened our conviction of the great role of elements in human health.

We propose a quadrilateral approach on which research has immense potentialities of development.

1. Elemental composition of human body in healthy subjects.
2. Changes in elemental composition in different diseases.
3. Determination of elements in simple and compound drugs.
4. Changes in body elements through the use of these drugs during disease states.

We are aware that these approaches, though easily enumerated, are very difficult in application. At the present state of knowledge, there appear to be two major hurdles: (*a*) wide variation in base line values and (*b*) lack of precision analytical equipment/techniques which are practicable in field conditions. The science of Medical Elementology is faced with more questions than can be answered today. Dedicated effort is warranted to put the possibilities to practical (diagnostic and therapeutic) applications.

BIOLOGICAL CLASSIFICATION OF ELEMENTS (VOHORA, 1989)

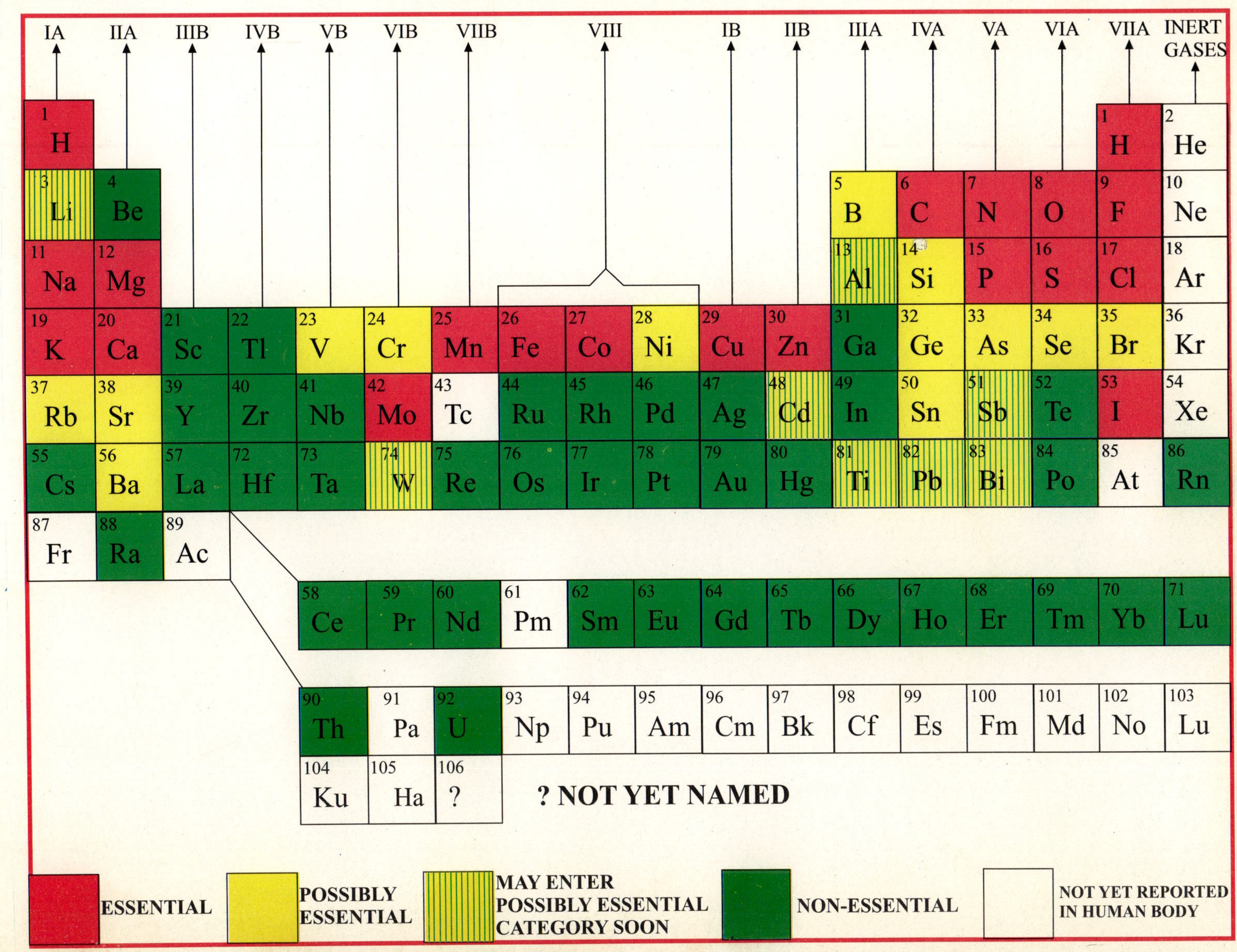

2

ELEMENTS

ACTINIUM (Ac)

CATEGORY

Not reported in human body.

ALUMINIUM (Al)

CATEGORY

Non-essential accumulative element. Some workers class it as a biostimulant.[59]

DISTRIBUTION IN ECOSYSTEM [15,35,50,118,208]

AIR	**Al ng/m³**
North America and Europe	1
WATER	**Al g/L**
Fresh water	1 - 50
The concentration increases with acidity	
SOIL	**Al g/kg**
Surface soil	71
Most abundant element in earth's crust	8%

PLANT FOODS [95,118]

	Al mg/kg f
Cereals	1.2 - 5.4
Potatoes	1.2 - 2.5
Vegetables	0.1 - 5.0
Fruits	0.4 - 2.8
Mushrooms	4.0
Tea	128.0
Coffee	30.5

ANIMAL FOODS [12,15,59,95,118]

	Al mg/kgf
Milk and Milk Products	0.8-2.0
Meat and Liver	5.0
Cooked Beef	0.2
Cooked Cod Fish	0.4

HUMAN BODY

Whole Body Content [158,210,211]

- 0.9 ppm
- Content in average adult man (60 kg) : 61 mg

Distribution [91,93,187,209,211]

- Widely distributed in more than 48 tissues and body fluids including all vital organ.

■ **Blood**	**Al µg/L**
Whole blood	170 - 720 (mean : 300)
Erythrocytes	64 - 4600
Serum	110 - 780 (mean : 280)

- **Tissues**

Wide range of values reported. Highest concentration in lungs which increases with age.

	Al µg/g ash
Lungs	2500 - 4500
Liver	65 - 500
Kidneys	35 - 560
Brain	13 - 360
Heart	30 - 310
Skin	400 - 1000

ROLE

No role/essentiality has been attributed to this element.

DEFICIENCY

No adverse effects were observed in goats given low Al semisynthetic ration (162 μg/kg for 4 years). While their food intake, growth, reproduction, and milk production was normal, the life expectancy of such goats was significantly reduced vs. control goats receiving 25 mg Al/kg.[209]

No report of any deficiency syndrome is available in human beings.

METABOLISM [118,209]

Absorption

While inhalatory absorption is the main cause of Al toxicity, absorption (< 1-2%) also takes place from the gastro-intestinal tract. Higher amounts may be absorbed orally from acidic diet and in pathological states, *e.g.*, chronic renal failure. Role of transferrin, Ca and parathyroid hormone has been speculated in absorption of orally ingested Al. Substantial inhalatory absorption has been reported following occupational exposure to Al dust, vapours and fumes. Acid rain may increase environmental availability of this metal.

Distribution and Metabolism

Significant retention takes place only at very high levels of intake *e.g.*, following administration of antacids. Distribution occurs to almost all tissues and body fluids with high concentrations in lungs, bones and muscles. It crosses both blood-brain and placental barriers. Aluminium interacts with and inhibits absorption of Ca, F, Fe, Mg and Sr.

Excretion

Excretion occurs through feces, bile, urine and exhaled air. Renal excretion is the main route following inhalatory exposure. Hyperaluminemia has been reported in oligouric and anuric patients suffering from chronic renal failure.

INTAKE/REQUIREMENTS [118,209]

Range of intake from Western Diets	3-14 Al mg/day
Tolerable weekly intake	7 mg/kg body weight

No RDA worked out as Al is not an essential element.

GUIDELINE VALUES [118]

	Al mg/m^3
Occupational exposure limit (OEL)	
(40 h work week)	2-10
OEL for Al metal oxide/hydroxide as fine dust or fumes	6
Drinking water	**Al mg/L**
(Permissible limit)	0.2
Biological exposure limit	**Al µg/L**
Plasma	10
Urine	200

MEDICINAL USES

Aluminium carbonate, phosphate and hydroxide gel are used in medicine (antacids) and cosmetics (antiperspirant talcs).[15,81,200] It has also been used to treat fluorosis and reduce phosphate absorption in uremic patients.[209]

TOXICITY

There is high degree of tolerance to this metal. At a dose of 10 ppm, administered in drinking water for life, no untoward effects were observed in rats and mice. Fatal doses in animals are quite high 5-10 g in cats, 35-50 g in dogs and 500 g in cattle. Evidence for toxicity in human beings is available in cases of impaired renal function and dialysis therapy.[145,209] It is considered as a potential neurotoxicant in men. Diseases associated with elevated Al levels include pulmonary fibrosis, renal osteodystrophy, bone disease linked with parentral nutrition, anaemia, cardiotoxicity, cancer and dialysis encephalopathy.[103] Significantly higher serum Al levels were reported in epileptic patients vs. control subjects.[192]

SOURCES OF EXPOSURE [15,50,118,209]

From household and industrial uses/contamination:

(*a*) Cooking utensils/cans

(*b*) Water for dialysis

(*c*) Pharmaceuticals (specially antacids) and cosmetics

(*d*) Construction material

(*e*) Transport vehicles/Aircraft and Rockets

(*f*) Electrical equipment/wires

(*g*) Packing material

(*h*) Grain fumigant

(*i*) Food additives

(*j*) Paint pigment etc.

SYSTEMIC EFFECTS [15,50,200,209]

These include gastro-intestinal disturbances, respiratory symptoms (metal fume fever, bronchitis, pulmonary fibrosis), disturbances in blood coagulation, anaemia, negative P balance with rickets and osteomalacia, encephalopathy, Alzheimer's disease and neurological lesions (when serum Al levels exceed 300 μg/L). Exposure to Al dextran and Al oxide dusts (particle size 1-5 micron) has been shown to cause lung oedema and cancer in experimental animals. Human evidence for carcinogenic effects is not available. Two distinct diseases have been reported following dialysis with water containing > 50 μg/L of Al either from natural source or when aluminium sulphate is added to precipitate particulate matter. These are **(*a*) Dialysis dementia** and **(*b*) Dialysis osteodystrophy** with symptoms of bone pain, speech disorder, loss of memory, dementia and myoclonus. The latter may be fatal. In a study on 258 patients on home dialysis (with water containing > 80 μg/L Al), 18 patients developed dementia. It is absolutely necessary to remove excess Al from water for safe dialysis, reverse osmosis is helpful in affected persons.

MECHANISM OF TOXICITY [15]

- Alterations in Ca and ferritin concentrations in brain
- Dephosphorylation of proteins *e.g.*, by complex formation with inositol phosphate leading to negative P balance.

TREATMENT

Chelation with Tiron, Desferrioxamine and Glutathione is useful for the treatment of Al poisoning.

ANTIMONY (Sb)

CATEGORY

Non-essential accumulative element

DISTRIBUTION IN ECOSYSTEM [35, 95, 118]

AIR	**Sb ng/m^3**
Chicago, USA	1.4 - 5.5
WATER	**Sb g/L**
Sea water	0.2
Fresh water	0.5 - 1.0
SOIL	**Sb ppm**
Earth's crust	0.2 - 0.3
Soil	4.3 - 8.0

PLANTS [95,118]

	Sb mg/kg (dry weight)
Tobacco	0.1

Trace amounts detected in some vegetables (*e.g.*, spinach), alfa alfa and algae

ANIMAL FOODS [12,15,118]

	Sb µg/kg wet weight
Milk	3.0
Fresh-water fish	3.0
Oyesters	< 0.7

HUMAN BODY

Whole Body Content [158,187,211]

- 0.9 ppm
- Content in average adult man (60 kg) : 61 mg

Distribution [93]

Presence has been detected in blood (3 g/L) and almost all tissues by neutron activation analysis (NAA) technique. Data available for content in 34 tissues and body fluids.

ROLE/ESSENTIALITY

There is no evidence for any role/essentiality of Sb for animals and human beings.

DEFICIENCY

No deficiency syndrome for this element is known.

METABOLISM [118]

Absorption

Oral absorption is very poor. Inhalatory absorption has been reported following occupational exposure to dust and fumes.

Distribution/Metabolism

Widely distributed with high retention in lungs, liver, kidneys, spleen, adrenal glands, skin, hair and lymph glands.

Excretion

Most of the ingested Sb is excreted unabsorbed in feces. Pentavalent Sb compounds are mainly excreted in urine and trivalent forms in feces.

INTAKE/REQUIREMENTS [209]

	Sb g/day
Intake	0.20 - 23 (Median : 2.6)

RDA values have not been worked out because Sb is a non-essential element.

GUIDELINE VALUES

	Sb mg/m^3
Occupational Exposure Limit (Germany)	0.2 - 2.0
Maximum Concentration for Stibine	0.5

MEDICINAL USES [195,200]

- Trivalent Sb compounds (*e.g.*, Sb potassium tartrate, stibophen etc.), earlier used for expectorant and emetic actions, are not used now because of high toxicity and availability of better drugs for such effects.
- Pentavalent antimonials (*e.g.*, Stibamine, Stibosan, Neostam etc.) occupy important place in the treatment of protozoal infections and helminth infections *e.g.*, leishmaniasis, trypanosomiasis, schistosomiasis and filariasis.
- Potential effect of an Sb compound (ammonium-5-tungsto-2-antimoniate), as reverse transkriptase inhibitor, can be explored for therapeutic utility:
  (*a*) against AID virus and (*b*) to facilitate increase in peripheral lymphocytes.
- Traditional eye cosmetics *Surma* are reported to have high content of Sb. Scientific reports to establish their therapeutic efficacy and mechanism(s) involved are not available.
- Some Sb derivatives *e.g.*, ^{203}Sb, tartrate and organic compounds have recently been reported to show interesting results in the treatment of cancer.[48]

TOXICITY [158,187,195]

Sources of Exposure

From industrial and other uses in:

(*a*) Mining of ores, stibnite, kermesite, valentinite, cervantite.

(*b*) Use of alloys in batteries, bearings, electronic industry (thermocouples and semiconductors).

(*c*) Fire works

(*d*) Ammunition

(*e*) Ceremics/glass works. Glazed pottery.

(*f*) Vulcanization of rubber.

(*g*) Parasiticidal drugs and other medicinal uses.

Poisoning

Poisoning may occur from occupational exposure (*e.g.*, in smelter operations where air concentrations may reach up to 10 mg/m^3), from food (specially acid food) in contact with enamelled utensils containing Sb oxide, and overdosage of parasiticidal agents. Trivalent Sb is more toxic vs. pentavalent form. Extensive human studies are not available. Findings from studies on experimental animals, *in vitro* studies in cell cultures and some human reports indicate Sb and stibine exert toxic effects on heart, liver, kidney, lungs, brain, bone marrow etc. Inhalatory exposure is particularly hazardous. It causes extensive pulmonary deposition, pneumonitis and pneumoconiosis. Stibine is reported to cause bone marrow damage, fibrosis, and toxic effects on erythrocytes and the nervous system. There is considerable evidence for mutagenic and carcinogenic actions of Sb. It has been linked to the incidence of carcinoma of lungs following chronic exposure at work place. A high incidence of urinary bladder tumours in patients with schistosomiasis is suspected to be caused by antimonials. Experimental studies revealed that prolonged administration of Sb shortened the life span of rats.

MECHANISM OF TOXICITY [47,195]

- Local irritation.
- Inhibition of SH group of essential enzymes.
- Potential to produce oxygen species and interference with DNA repair system.

TREATMENT

- Chelation with Unithiol (5% solution, 0.1 ml/kg i.m., 3 - 4 times on Day 1 followed by 2-3 times on Day 2 and 1-2 times on Days 3-7). Children 5 - 10 years are given 1/3 to 1/2 of the adult dose.
- Symptomatic therapy includes alkali inhalations, gargles, ephedrine/adrenaline, drinking of warm sweet tea, tannin solution, milk etc.

ARGON (Ar)

CATEGORY

Inert gas, not reported in human body.

ARSENIC (As)

CATEGORY

- Possibly essential ultra-trace element
- With an atomic number of 33, it falls within the critical range of essentiality (23 to 34)

DISTRIBUTION IN ECOSYSTEMS [35,50,118]

As in nature is mainly bound to S : arsenopyrite and orpiment.

AIR

	As ng/m^3
Remote Areas (Greenland)	0.007

North America	2 - 40
Europe	1.5 - 53
India	NA
WATER	**As μg/kg**
River water	1.7
Sea water	1.6

Groundwater: As gets mobilized into it from soil under acidic conditions. Consumption and use of such water should be restricted to protect public health. Well water in South India, Kolkata and Bangladesh contains high levels of As (upto 3.7 mg/L). Ministry of Health, Government of India considers a level of 0.2 mg/L to be excessive.

SOIL

Surface soil	**As conc. mg/kg**
Mean	8
Range	0.7-30

PLANTS [12,118]

Bioaccumulation index

Plant : Soil ratio	0.01 to 0.1
Concentration at which no sensitivity develops in immature plants	5 - 20 mg/kg

Food plants

		As mg/kg fresh weight
Low 30-70 μg/kg	Cereals (wheat, rice, rye)	0.05
	Potatoes	0.07
	Vegetables (lettuce, cabbage, celery,: tomatoes, spinach, cucumber)	0.03 - 0.04
	Fruits (peaches, bananas, apples, citrus fruits)	0.02 - 0.04
High 132-320 μg/kg high	Mushrooms	0.14
	Tea	0.13
	Coffee	0.32

Raddish and tobacco are rich in As content. Fruits and vegetables sprayed with arsenical pesticides/herbicides may acquire high As concentration.

ANIMALS [12,15,118]

Wild animals	
Whole body weight	0.4 to 1.1 ppm
Animal foods	**mg/kg fresh wt.**
Meat, Pork, Chicken, Beef	0.01 to 6.3
Higher content in Organ Meats : Liver, Kidney	upto 10 to 15

Sometimes added to poultry feed to stimulate growth. This may lead to high As content in chicken.

Milk	< 50 μg/L

Sea food

Relatively rich in As content but it is present in stable non-toxic forms eg:

Arsenobetaine

Arsenocholine

Arsenolecithin

	mg/kg fresh weight
Marine fish	1-10
Prawns	upto 175
Mussels	upto 120
Oyesters:	upto 3.7

MICROORGANISMS

- Paints/pigments containing As undergo biomethylation by the action of moulds yielding a gas with garlic-like odour.
- Methylated forms of As are observed in natural waters.
- Biomethylating organisms:

  Candida lumicola

  Methanobacter

HUMAN BODY [93,158,187,211]

Whole Body Content

- 1.1×10^{20} atoms in the body
- 1.1×10^{6} atoms in each cell
- 0.2 ppm
- Content in an average adult man (60 Kg): approx. 14 mg.

Distribution

- Distributed in > 25 human tissues and body fluids including all vital organs, brain, heart, liver, lungs, kidneys, pancreas, spleen, thyroid, adrenals, ovary, prostate, placenta, uterus, blood, milk, bones, skin, lymph glands etc.
- Predilection for fat. Associated with lipid phase of brain tissue.

	As µg/g
Brain, heart, liver, kidneys, lungs	0.01-0.05
Skin	0.09-0.12
Blood plasma	2.4-10.0 µg/L

ROLE/ESSENTIALITY [59]

- Precise role is not known.
- Indicators are available to suggest:
  - (*a*) It takes part in reactions involving phosphate groups,
  - (*b*) Plays a structural role as part of membrane phospholipids,
  - (*c*) Influences metabolism of : arginine, methionine, zinc and labile methyl groups,
  - (*d*) Catalyzes glutathione biosynthesis,
  - (*e*) Can both activate and inhibit enzymes *in vitro*

DEFICIENCY [1,2,4,59]

- Experimental deficiency in animals (rats, minipigs, chicks, goats) given totally arsenic-free diets, leads to signs of deprivation:
  - (*i*) depressed growth.
  - (*ii*) impaired reproduction (decreased fertility and increased pup mortality).
  - (*iii*) rough skin/feathers.
  - (*iv*) sudden death during lactation (myocardial damage).

- Dietary supplementation reverses signs and symptoms of deficiency.
- Human deficiency has not been reported. Low serum As levels have, however, been shown in hemodialysis patients. Low As levels are also observed in CNS diseases.

METABOLISM [15,50,58,118,209]

Absorption

It depends on:

(*i*) **Type of Compound : Solubility and Physical form**

– Oxides are poorly soluble and so are poorly absorbed.

– Inorganic arsenic forms are more readily absorbed vs. organic arsenicals (linked to a C atom with a covalent bond).

(*ii*) **Route of administration:**

(*a*) ***Oral***

– There is high gastro-intestinal absorption for both trivalent and pentavalent As. Absorption for soluble forms : 70-90%.

– Arsine gas is most readily absorbed and is most toxic.

– Toxicity is in the following order :

Organic arsenicals $< A_s^{5+} < A_s^{3+} <$ Arsine gas
(Least toxic) (Most toxic)

(*b*) ***Cutaneous***

While absorption for pentavalent form is more vs. trivalent form by oral route, the absorption through skin is more for trivalent form.

(*c*) ***Inhalation***

Particle size is also a determinant.

Finer particles penetrate deeper into lung alveoli; coarse particles are caught in the upper respiratory tract.

Pulmonary absorption of soluble forms (*e.g.*, As trioxide) is rapid. Less soluble forms (*e.g.*, Ca and Pb arsenate) reside in lower airways for long and are absorbed slowly.

Distribution/Metabolism

- Binding occurs with SH groups and globin part of hemoglobin in erythrocytes (95-99%).
- Half life : 60-80 days.
- Bound form transported to other tissues (liver, kidneys, lungs, heart etc.) and body fluids within 24 hours. Longest retention for dimethyl arsenic acid is reported in lungs, thyroid and lens of the eye.

- Deposition in 2 weeks in bones, nails and skin. It persists in these tissues for years.
- Deposition in bones because of role in phosphate groups and in skin/nails because of affinity for keratin. Binding with keratin in hair, nails and skin is particularly strong.
- Crosses both blood-brain and placental barriers.
- Interacts with Se and protects against Se toxicity.

Detoxification

- Trivalent form $\xrightarrow[\text{in blood}]{\text{Reduction}}$ Pentavalent form
- Biomethylation by methanobacteria (enzymatic transfer of methyl group from S-adenosyl methionine). This leads to formation of:
  – Monomethyl arsonic acid (MMAA)

  and

  – Dimethyl arsinic acid (DMAA)
- These reactions are catalysed by methyltransferase (s) with S-adenosyl-methionine as cofactor and glutathione as reducer.

Excretion

- 70-80% of ingested As is excreted in urine. Organic arsenicals of low solubility (*e.g.*, in sea food) are readily excreted and are least toxic.

  Half life : 3-5 days,

  Major forms : (*a*) Cacodylic acid and Methanearsonic acid in man.

  (*b*) Arsenobetaine and Arsenolipids in aquatic organisms.
- Excretion also occurs through feces, skin, hair, sweat, breath and milk.
- Urine analysis for DMAA constitutes a reliable index for rate of clearance or degree of accumulation/toxicity.

For example :

	Children urine Concentration in μg/g
Non-smoking parents	4.2
One parent smoking	5.5
Both parents smoking	13.0

INTAKE

	µg per day
Infants 0 - 6 months	25-51
Adults	10-300

Dietary intake of approx. 3 mg/day for 2-3 weeks causes toxicity. Contaminated drinking water, rather than its dietary intake, is the cause of chronic As poisoning in human beings.[209]

REQUIREMENTS

- No known requirements. Too much refining of foods may lead to deficiency syndrome in future.
- In a German scientific conference, one of the questions was: Are people getting enough As in diet?
- Nielsen[133] described it to be an essential nutrient for animals.

Estimated requirements	< 50 ng/g of diet
	6.25-12.5 µg/1000 KCal
Human values calculated from animal data	15-25 µg/day

GUIDELINE VALUE [15,118,209]

- Drinking water

Permissible (WHO)	10 µg/l*
Excessive (India)	0.2 mg/l

*This may, however, lead to excess lifetime intake levels and risk of skin cancer.

■ Occupational exposure limit (OEL in air on 40 h work week)	0.2 mg/m³
■ Urine As	15-40 µg/l
■ Hair As	< 1 µg/g
■ Maximum concentration of Arsine gas at work place.	0.05 ppm
■ Technical guideline concentration for As compounds in total dust.	0.2 mg/m³
■ Soil As	< 20 mg/kg

- Sodium arsenite banned as herbicide in many countries.
- Listed by EP under hazardous waste category.

MEDICINAL USES

Indian systems of medicine (Ayurveda, Siddha and Unani-Tibb) use even such metals for medicinal purposes which are otherwise considered toxic. These are used in calcined forms incorporating herbal juices during the ashing process. Traditional calcined preparations of As *e.g.*, *Hartal Bhasma, Kushta Hartal Warqi* and *Kushta Samm-ul-Far* have been attributed with diverse medicinal/therapeutic properties including general tonic, aphrodisiac, anti-rheumatic, anti-catarrhal, anti-asthmatic, anti-diabetic properties and utility in fevers, gout, leprosy, tremors, epilepsy, general and facial paralysis.[5,8,126,154,160] Most of these claims have not been investigated. Some recent studies revealed interesting analgesic, anti-cataleptic, anxiolytic glycogen sparing (anti-fatigue) and growth promoting effects in *Kushta Hartal* and *Kushta Sammu-ul-Far* without discernible toxicity in rodents under normal conditions.

Qawi and *Aatishaki* varieties of *Kushta Sammul Far* (5mg Kg^{-1} po for 10 days) did not produce significant biochemical (Serum AST, ALT, Creatinine and Urea concentrations) and histopathological (brain, liver and kidneys) alterations in rats. Some pro-convulsant potential (reduction in various phases of convulsions and mortality in pentylene tetrazol and maximal eletroshock models) was, however, detected which is quite disturbing and calls for caution.[63,64,167-171] One clinical study reported the efficacy and tolerability of *Kushta Hartal* (Tabqi) in cases of maturity onset diabetes mellitus.[151] This is an isolated report. No other study to confirm or refute these findings is available.

It is interesting to note that As is now under investigation for anticancer activity.[165] Arsenic trioxide is now approved for the treatment of promyocytic leukemia and is under investigation for several other malignancies (*e.g.*, multiple myeloma, cutaneous lymphoma, cystic tumours etc.) in China, Europe, Canada and USA. [37,87,106,165,166,204,215]

Waxman and Anderson[205] reviewed history and development of the use of As derivatives in cancer.

TOXICITY [15,50]

- Arsenic is considered 'King of poisons'. Soluble inorganic salts are highly toxic. Lethal dose of ingested As trioxide : 1-3 mg/kg body weight.
- It is odourless and tasteless and so can be mixed in food and drinks undetected. Used for homicidal and suicidal purposes.

SOURCES OF EXPOSURE/CONTAMINATION [15,50,187,209]

From extensive usage and contamination:

(*a*) Pesticides

(*b*) Herbicides

(*c*) Rodenticides

(*d*) Glass and ceramic works

(*e*) Geo-thermal power plant effluents

(*f*) Gallium arsenide in electronic industry

(*g*) Earlier organic arsenicals were used as chemotherapeutic agents in trypanosomiasis

(*h*) Uses in traditional medicines: Ayurveda and Unani-Tibb.

(*i*) Well water in certain areas.

SYSTEMIC EFFECTS [1,4,15,48,50,118,181,188,190,209,215,216,219]

1. ***Liver:*** Hepatotoxic in man and animals. Poisoning commonly results from insecticides/rodenticides and adulterated opium. Chronic poisoning observed in regions with high As content in ground water. Some vegetables e.g. onions and radish accumulate large concentration of As in these regions. Industrial/occupational exposure causes cirrhosis, fatty infiltration, central necrosis, bile duct thrombosis and hepatic cancer. High As concentrations are observed in liver in all cirrhotic diseases including alcoholic cirrhosis and Indian childhood cirrhosis.

2. ***GIT:*** The symptoms include epigastric pain, colic, gradual splanchnic hyperemia, diarrhoea, sloughing of mucus membranes, rice water stools, blood in feces and vomitus.

3. ***Kidneys:*** Renal toxicity in man and animals. Experimental toxicity has been produced in rabbits. Arsenic causes tubular damage/necrosis. Patients with uremia show high tissue As levels in kidneys, muscles, liver, spleen, lungs etc. Toxicity is manifested by oligourea, proteinuria and hematuria. Urine shows presence of hemoglobin and casts. Arsine gas causes severe damage. Urinary As concentrations constitute a good index of intoxication.

4. ***Nervous system:*** Peripheral neuropathy (both motor and sensory) is the key feature of effects on nervous system. Besides there may be dysthesia, decrease in deep tendon reflexes, muscular weakness, muscular atrophy etc.

5. ***Cardiovascular system:*** Arsenic is a capillary poison. It affects oxidative enzymes, causes hypovolemia which may result in fatal hypovolemic shock with circulatory failure. Other signs and symptoms include oedema, increase in body weight, hypotension, anaemia, leucopenia, basophilic stippling, myocarditis, ECG changes (*e.g.*, increased QT interval, T wave inversion), hemolysis, hemoglobin in urine, splanching of face, chronic bone marrow depression, low blood folic acids levels and Renaud's syndrome.

6. ***Respiratory system:*** Occupational inhalatory exposure in grape garden sprayers may lead to acute, sub-acute or chronic toxicity with inflammation of the mucus membranes of the respiratory tract. This is manifested by corhyza, tracheobronchitis, cough, perforation of nasal septum, epistaxis, pneumonitis with high incidence of cancer.

7. ***Skin:*** Hyperpigmentation/melanosis is a common manifestation with hyperkeratoses of palms and soles. Black foot disease, rain drop rash and high incidence of squamous cell carcinoma are observed in areas with high As content in water.

8. ***Immune Functions:*** A biphasic effect is observed. Low doses cause proliferation of T cells and increased formation of antibody forming cells in response to mitogens and heterologous antigens. High doses, on the other hand, elicit immunosuppressive effect.

9. ***Carcinogenic Effect:*** Arsenic presents the anomaly of displaying both anti-cancer and oncogenic properties. Conflicting reports are available on the carcinogenic potential (or otherwise) of arsenic. Epidemiological studies indicate an association of As with skin and lung cancers. The time lag between exposure and effect may be as long as 70 years. Sodium arsenite has, therefore, been banned in many countries for use as a herbicide. According to a WHO study exposure of workers to 0.25 μg/m^3 As in air for 25 years, lead to 10% higher incidence of lung cancer. A recent Polish study established a positive co-relation between urine As concentrations and some neoplastic markers.

The ambient air in Prague contains high levels of As tri-oxide. It is argued that if As is carcinogenic, at such exposure levels, it should result in high incidence (in epidemic proportions) of lung cancer in this region but it is not so. According to another report from USA, people getting well water with high As content, exhibited better health records vs. general population. Animal experiments to induce cancer with As alone have not been always successful. Moreover long-term feeding of arsenicals in experimental animals, resulted in less incidence of breast and lung cancers. But rodent cells are known to be less susceptible to cancer induction vs. human cells. It may be concluded that As can, at worst, be a promoter (rather than an initiator) of cancer.

There is renewed interest in the therapeutic utility of arsenic following reports of the use of arsenic trioxide in the treatment of cancer especially leukemia.

10. ***Teratogenic Effects:*** Arsenic acts as a co-mutagen in the presence of chemical mutagens and UV light. Sodium arsenite and arsenate have been reported to cross the placental barrier and cause teratogenic effects. While malformations of the brain, urinogenital organs, skeleton and eye have been reported following high exposure to As during fetal development in experimental animals, human data for such effects are lacking.

MECHANISMS OF TOXICITY [15,50,118]

(*a*) As impairs cellular respiration through interaction with mitochondrial enzymes *e.g.*, succinic dehydrogenase and cofactors *e.g.*, dihydrolipoic acid.

(*b*) Pentavalent As is an uncoupler of oxidative phosphorylation. The effect is competitive resulting in substitution of arsenate for inorganic PO_4 in ATP and formation of an arsenate ester. The latter is rapidly hydrolyzed : arsenolysis.

(*c*) Trivalent As reacts with available SH-ligands. Pyruvate dehydrogenase group is specially sensitive because interaction occurs with two SH groups of lipoic acid with formation of six-member stable rings.

(*d*) Induction of apoptosis in T lymphoma cells: partially caspase-independent pathway.

(*e*) Inhibition of heme synthesis through inhibition of heme synthetase and δ ALA synthetase enzymes.

(*f*) Axon-sensitive degeneration.

(*g*) Enhancement of lipid peroxidation.

(*h*) Hypovolemia.

DIAGNOSTIC FEATURES [15,50,118]

Symptoms are observed within 30 min, death occurs in 1-12 hours.

(*i*) Severe epigastric pain, metallic taste, dry mouth, constriction in throat.

(*ii*) Rice water stools.

(*iii*) Oligourea, anuria or hematuria and blood in vomitus.

(*iv*) Leg cramps, tingling in limbs, ataxia.

(*v*) Hyperpigmentation of skin, mucus membranes, extremities

(*vi*) Black foot disease, Rain drop rash

(*vii*) Paralysis, irrational speech.

(*viii*) Hemolytic anemia followed renal failure in cases of arsine gas poisoning.

TREATMENT

- Chelation indicated when urine As levels are > 200 µg/L.
- Choice of Agents :

  First choice : DMPS, DMSA

  Second choice : Dimercaprol or BAL
- Also useful are unithiol, dicaptol, dithioglyceral, sodium thiosulphate and ascorbic acid.
- Hemodialysis is required if there is danger of renal failure.
- In cases of poisoning with Arsine gas, if free hemoglobin level is > 1.5 g/100 ml, exchange transfusion can be given.
- The patients should be monitored for complications and symptomic therapy given for anaemia, ECG changes, liver and pulmonary function abnormalities and K loss.

ASTATINE (At)

CATEGORY

Not reported in human body.

BARIUM (Ba)

CATEGORY

Possibly essential ultra trace element

DISTRIBUTION IN ECOSYSTEM

- Detailed reports are not available.
- Toxic metal is mobilized into ground water under acidic conditions..

HUMAN BODY [36,93,158,195,210,211]

Whole Body Content

- 0.3 ppm
- Content in average adult man (60 kg) : 23.8 mg

Distribution

Distributed in > 45 tissues and body fluids including all vital organs. Relatively higher content in lungs, aorta and eyes vs. other tissues. The content increases with age.

Blood	
Whole blood	01. µg/g wet wt.
Tissues	**Ba µg/g ash**
Heart	7.4
Brain	2.6
Liver	3.5
Lungs	9.9

ROLE/ESSENTIALITY [118,158,176]

- Inspite of its wide distribution, the role Ba is not known.
- Some workers consider it to be a non-essential/accumulative element while others describe it as an essential element (it can spare Ca).
- Omission from mineral supplements of rats and guinea pigs has been reported to cause growth depression.
- Constant presence in pigmented parts of the eye was stated to be an unresolved mystery of human body composition.

DEFICIENCY

No deficiency syndrome has been reported both in animals and man.

METABOLISM [118,187]

Detailed studies are not available. Gastrointestinal absorption is reported to be as follows:

Insoluble salts	< 1%
Soluble salts	10-30%

Bulk of excretion takes place through feces (unabsorbed part + some secreted back into gastrointestinal tract). Excretion also occurs via urine sweat and hairs. It has been postulated that phagocytosis of Ba (II) may be an important route of entry into mammalian cell.

INTAKE/REQUIREMENTS

Variable Ba intake values ranging between 592 to 750 μg/day have been reported. As its essentiality is not known, requirements have not been worked out.

GUIDELINE VALUES [118]

Ba mg/m^3

Soluble compounds	0.5

Listed by EP in hazardous waste category

MEDICINAL USES [187,194]

- Insoluble salt $BaSO_4$ is extensively used in X-ray as an opaque contrast for diagnostic purposes.
- Used for local effects around cement fixed prostheses.
- Older use of $BaCl_2$ in Stoke Adam's disease has been discontinued because of doubtful efficacy and high toxicity.
- $BaCl_2$ has been used for precipitation and removal of ^{226}Ra in mine water ponds and U industry.

TOXICITY [15,77,195,200]

Sources

- Barium ion is one of the most toxic elements of alkaline earth series.
- Barium carbonate (used as a rodenticide) is a white powder frequently mistaken for flour.

- It is considered a hazardous waste. Damage from dumping waste and in landfills has been reported in USA.
- The metal has been listed among 8 metals specified in EP toxicity tests for hazardous industrial contaminants.
- Ba gets mobilized into groundwater under acidic conditions. Consumption and use of such water should be restricted to protect public health.

Effects

- Ba gets accumulated in bones on prolonged exposure displacing Ca with adverse effects.
- It exerts a direct stimulant action on all smooth muscles causing powerful contractions of the entire gastrointestinal tract. The symptoms include nausea, vomiting, severe abdominal pain and diarrhoea.
- Barium acts as a hepatotoxin causing fatty liver. Lower blood Ba levels have been reported in cases of hepatic cirrhosis, choleocystitis and primary carcinoma of liver.
- Barium compounds produce neuromuscular blockade by persistent depolarization at the neuromuscular junction.
- Toxic effects on other systems are bronchoconstriction, pneumoconiasis (by Badust), hypertention, palpitation, extrasystoles, paralysis etc.
- Ingestion of 1g of a soluble salt may be fatal.

BERYLLIUM (Be)

CATEGORY

Non-essential accumulative trace element.

DISTRIBUTION IN ECOSYSTEM [15,35,118]

AIR	**Be ng/m³**
USA	< 0.1-6.7
Europe	2.0
Japan	0.04-0.2
WATER	**Be mg/m³**
Sea water	0.006
Freshwater	0.3
Higher content in acid lakes (upto 1-2 μg/L)	
SOIL	**Be mg/kg**
Surface soil	1-7

PLANT FOODS [15,118]

Plants contain only trace amounts of Be except when grown in Be rich culture solutions with following values in edible plants:

	Be ppm
Potatoes	0.17
Tomatoes	0.24
Peas	upto 75
Cloves	18-22
Fruits	< 4
Polished rice	0.08

Terrestrial plants contain < 1 mg/kg Be (dry weight)

ANIMAL FOODS [12,92,118]

	Be μg/kg
Milk and milk products	< 0.75
Mammalian muscle	0.75
Salt water fish	2-200

HUMAN BODY [9,93,118,187,208,209]

Whole Body Content

- 0.001 ppm
- Content in average adult man (60 kg) : 36 μg

Distribution

Reported present in more than 11 tissues and body fluids

Blood

Whole blood	< 0.1-3.8 μg/L

Tissues

High content in liver, lungs, skin and bone

	Be μg/100 g
Liver	0.012
Lungs	0.23

ROLE/ESSENTIALITY [6,9,15,195]

Beryllium is a non-essential element. It has not been attributed with any role/function in animals and man.

DEFICIENCY

No deficiency syndrome has been reported for this element.

METABOLISM [6,9,15,195]

Detailed studies are not available. Gastrointestinal absorption is very poor (0.01%). However soluble salts may be absorbed upto 20%. Some cutaneous absorption has also been reported. Substantial absorption takes place through the inhalatory route. The latter is mainly responsible for its toxic effects following occupational exposure. The metal is transported through blood in colloidal form (phosphate or hydroxide complexes). There is greater retention in liver, lungs reticuloendothelial system and skeleton. Bulk of the ingested Be is excreted unabsorbed in feces. Inhaled Be is excreted through urine, hair and sweat and some part is retained in lungs. Pulmonary excretion is biphasic: phase-1 is fast during first 1-2 weeks after cessation of exposure, phase-2 is slow.

INTAKE/REQUIREMENTS [195]

Daily intake from food, water and air is 13 μg. The element is not required for animals and man.

GUIDELINE VALUES [15,118]

	Be μg/m^3 Air
Occupational Exposure Limit (40 hour work week)	2

Be is classified as a carcinogen. European community prohibits its use in cosmetics.

Single Determination Value	25
Community Air (One Month Average)	0.01

MEDICINAL USES

Be is not used for any medicinal purpose.

TOXICITY [6,9,15,42,50,118,195]

Sources of Exposure

From industrial/personal uses in:

(*a*) Electrical contacts

(*b*) Insulators for power transistors

(*c*) Sparklers tools and Bearing shells

(*d*) Telecommunication

(*e*) Colouring gemstones

(*f*) Ceramics

(*g*) Dental alloys

(*h*) Nuclear reactors/Atomic energy installations

(*i*) Rockets

(*j*) Radars

(*k*) Space vehicle etc.

While administration of Be, 5 ppm in drinking water produces toxic effects in experimental animals, the metal is unlikely to cause toxicity by oral ingestion in man. Inhalatory exposure (Be > 100 μg/m^3 air) is a major occupational health problem. Principle toxic effects are on the respiratory system, skin, immune function, carcinogenicity and genotoxicity.

SYSTEMIC EFFECTS [9,15,50,195]

1. ***Liver:*** Acute toxicity is manifested by parenchymal hepatic necrosis in the median lobe. The toxin is reliberated by Kupffer cells causing further damage to liver cells.

2. ***Cardiovascular system:*** Hemopoietic function is adversely affected particularly in pregnant women.

3. ***Respiratory system:*** Massive inhalatory exposure causes acute Be disease/pneumonia which may be fatal. Chronic Be exposure over prolonged periods is manifested by reduced pulmonary function, dyspnoea, bronchitis, cough, interstitial pneumonitis, alveolar interstitial edema, miliary nodulation, fibrosis pneumosclerosis, lung cancer and granulomatous crippling. Both acute and chronic Be diseases has been reported in occupationally exposed persons. Chronic Be disease has a wide range latent period (several weeks to > 20 years) and is of long duration and severity. It has been proposed that a genetic modification of the major histocompatibility complex allele HLA-DPBl may be used as a biomarker of susceptibility to chronic Be disease.

4. ***Skin:*** Direct contact with skin causes contact dermatitis within a few days. Allergic eczematous reactions, ulcers and granulomas have also been reported following repeated exposure or contact with eroded skin/wounds. Healing of such ulcers does not take place until Be is completely removed from the wounds.

5. ***Reproductive system:*** Women are more susceptible to Be toxicity vs. males. It crosses placental barrier and is a potent toxicant to reproductive system causing no fetal resorption but high fetal mortality. Pregnancy apparently acts as a stress factor for Be toxicity.

6. ***Immune function:*** Alveolar clearance rate and macrophage phagocytic activity is reduced. Toxic effects on skin and respiratory system may be immunologically mediated. The metal induces hypersensitivity skin reactions and prevents wound healing. Chronic exposure to Be has been reported to (*a*) increase immunoglobulin levels, (*b*) depress sensitivity to tuberculin and (*c*) interfere with patch testing. The latter can not be used as a predictive test for Be hypersensitivity as the metal may itself induce sensitization reactions.

7. ***Carcinogenicity:*** It has been classified as a carcinogen by the International Agency for Research on Cancer (IARC). Both experimental and epidemiological evidence exists for the mutagenic and carcinogenic effects of Be. Pulmonary tumours were induced in rats and high incidence of various types of cancers was reported following chronic Be exposure. These include lung cancer, granulomas and osteogenic sarcomas.

8. ***Genotoxicity:*** The metal elicits genotoxic effects. It gets selectively bound to regulatory non-histone nuclear proteins, inhibits phosphatase enzymes, interferes with gene transcription and inhibits DNA synthesis (*in vitro* and *in vivo*).

MECHANISM OF TOXICITY [15,118]

- Inhibition of:
  - Magnesium
  - Enzymes involved in DNA synthesis, and catalysis of energy processes.
  - Phosphorylation reactions
- Immunotoxic, genotoxic and carcinogenic actions (described above).
- Increased lipid peroxidation.
- Local irritation and allergic reactions.

DIAGNOSTIC FEATURES [9]

- Respiratory and skin symptoms
- X-ray
- Blood lymphocyte proliferation test for Be sensitization.

TREATMENT [9]

- Chelation therapy is ineffective in removing Be^{2+} from tissues.
- Aurinnitrocarboxylic acid and Tiron.
- Symptomatic therapy using corticosteroids, bronchospasm arresting drugs, analeptics, oxygen etc.

BISMUTH (Bi)

CATEGORY

Non-essential accumulative trace element

DISTRIBUTION IN ECOSYSTEM [12,92,118]

Detailed reports are not available. The contents are very low in sea water, plants and animals. The latter has been partly attributed to low gastrointestinal absorption.

	Bi μg/kg
Earth's crust	< 200
Plants	60
Animals	
Land	4
Marine	10

HUMAN BODY [36,93,209]

Whole Body Content

- 0.3 ppm
- Content in average adult man (60 kg) : 200 μg

Distribution

The metal has been detected in 41 tissues and body fluids.

Blood

Whole blood	< 10 μg/L

Tissues

Accumulation was reported in some organs in the following order : Kidney, Liver, Spleen, Bones, Lungs, Heart and Muscles. The content in vital organs and skin is < 2 μg/g dry weight.

ROLE/ESSENTIALITY

No role or essential function is so far known for Bi. Some workers class it as a biostimulant.[59]

DEFICIENCY

No Bi deficiency syndrome has been reported.

METABOLISM [118,187]

Absorption from gastro intestinal tract is very poor (0.2-0.3%) and slow. Intestinal microflora appear to be important for Bi absorption. Bulk of the ingested Bi is excreted in feces (total in 8 days).

Binding occurs with a low molecular weight protein (other than metallothionein). Maximum retention was reported in kidneys which show Bi containing inclusion bodies. The absorbed fraction shows peak plasma levels within 15-60 min. of oral intake. It gets widely distributed including brain as the blood brain barrier is limited. Excretion occurs mainly in urine.

INTAKE/REQUIREMENTS [118]

	Bi μg/day
Intake through food and water	20

As it is a non-essential element, RDA values have not been worked out.

MEDICINAL USES [48,50,195,200]

- Sometimes used as contrast media for X-ray.
- Treatment of gastric ulcers (Bi subcitrate)
- Used in cosmetics (Bi oxide and sulphide)
- Earlier use of trivalent Bi compounds for the treatment of syphilis, diarrhoea, amoebiasis, burns etc. has been discontinued in favour of more effective and safe agents now available.
- Bi directly affects *Helicobacter pylori* and gastric lymphoma. Some Bi complexes of 6-mercaptopurine are promising anti-cancer agents.

TOXICITY

Sources of Exposure [15,71,77, 200]

From personal and industrial uses in:

(*a*) Semiconductors

(*b*) Cathodes in batteries

(*c*) Catalysts in petrochemical and heavy organic biochemical industries.

(*d*) Preparation and recycling of nuclear fuels.

(*e*) Pharmaceuticals and cosmetics (creams, dusting powders, hair dyes, tints/colouring, pearling agent in lipstics, freckle removers etc.)

Systemic Effects

Poisoning may occur following therapeutic use of Bi preparations.

(*a*) ***Gastro-intestinal systems:*** Patients with encephalopathy had constipation and those without encephalopathy exhibited colon disease and diarrhoea. Other symptoms include gingivitis and stomatitis indicating damage to oral mucosa. Nausea and vomiting have also been reported.

(*b*) ***Liver:*** Excess accumulation and hepatic damage occurs after large or repeated doses.

(*c*) ***Central Nervous System:*** Most prominent effects are on the CNS. Blood Bi levels > 170 μg/L were found to be associated with encephalopathy with symptoms of confusion, motor disturbances and treamours. The symptoms were manifested following high doses (0.7-20g/day) or prolonged therapy (4 weeks to 30 years) of Bi subnitrate or Bi subgallate and were mostly reversible (subsided following discontinuation of therapy).

(*d*) ***Kidney:*** Nephropathic effects (renal tubular damage and necrosis) may occur after Bi administration.

(*e*) ***Skin:*** Pigmentation (Melanosis) is commonly observed in patients under Bi therapy.

(*f*) ***Skeletal system:*** Accumulation in bones may be manifested by arthrosis.

(*g*) ***Blood:*** Methamoglobinemia.

MECHANISM OF TOXICITY

- Precise mechanism (s) involved are not known.
- Bi attacks SH group of essential enzymes.

TREATMENT

Dimercaprol is a useful antidote.

BORON (B)

CATEGORY

Possibly essential trace element.

DISTRIBUTION IN ECOSYSTEM

Not available

PLANT AND ANIMAL FOODS

Newnham[130,131] stated that it is impossible to remain alive on a B-free diet because it is present in all life-sustaining foods. Plant foods contain higher amounts of B vs. animal origin food items. Green vegetables, fruits, nuts and legumes are rich in B content particularly when grown without fertilizers. Bee pollen and some honys are also good sources. Animal products (meat, fish and dairy products) have low B content but colostrum contains approximately twice the amount of B present in milk.

HUMAN BODY [93,118,158,209,211]

Whole Body Content

- 0.7 ppm
- 0.37 mg/kg of fat-free tissues.
- Content in average adult man (60 kg): 48 mg.

Distribution

The element is reported present in at least 39 human tissues and body fluids including vital organs and skeleton suggesting wide distribution.

Blood	**B mg/L**
Whole blood	0.04 - 0.74
Plasma	0.12
Tissues	**B μg/g**
Bones	8.2
Brain, heart, kidneys, liver, lungs	0.05 - 0.6

ROLE/ESSENTIALITY 30,45,65,33-135

- In spite of wide distribution, the role of B in body is not precisely known. Only fragmentary information is available on its biochemical function in animal and human tissues.
- In 1923, B was found to be essential for plants (growth and cell division). Between 1923 and as late as 1980, the students of biology were taught that B was unique because it was essential for plants but not for animals and man. As late as in 1976, Schroeder stated that B is not needed for mammals. Since 1981, findings from animal experiments indicated that B may be of nutritional importance to higher animals including human beings.
- The status of B in plants has been equated with that of Si in animals. Both these elements are linked to stabilization of saccharides in connective tissue.
- It influences metabolism of (*a*) macrominerals, (*b*) electrolytes, (*c*) energy substrate, (*d*) nitrogen and (*e*) steroid hormones *e.g.*, parathyroid hormone.
- Effect is also reported on oxidative metabolism with elevation in erythrocyte SOD and serum ceruloplasmin levels and thereby on erythropoiesis.
- Two hypotheses have been proposed: (*a*) It is a negative regulator that influences a number of metabolic pathways by competitive inhibition of key enzyme systems and (*b*) Involvement in cell membrane function (structure, stability, transmembrane signalling or movement of regulatory cations or anions).
- It is believed to be essential for normal bone maintenance and joint function. Hydroxylases (which are responsible for transformation of Vitamins D_2 and D_3 into corresponding 1,2,5 dihydroxy derivatives) depend on borate ions.; Hence, B may be a potent protective factor against post-menopausal osteoporosis in women.

DEFICIENCY 45,133-135,209

- Variable symptoms (nature and severity) have been reported in animal studies. Attempts to induce deficiency in rats with diets containing only 155-163 ng/g B were not successful. Dietary content of Al, Ca, Mg, K, cholecalciferol, methionine etc. influence B deficiency syndrome, plasma/organ Ca and Mg concentrations, alkaline phosphatase and bone calcification. Response of experimental animals is enhanced by concurrent Mg deficiency and Al toxicity.

- Human deficiency has been linked to arthritis. Data from 13 countries revealed a negative correlation between boron content in soil, average daily intake and prevalence of arthritis in native population. Two examples are given below:

Country	Content in soil (ppm)	Average daily intake (mg)	Prevalence arthritis (%)
Jamaica	0.5	< 1	70
Israel	>2.5	10	1

Further B content in arthritic femur head (29.6 ppm) was found to be lower vs. that in normal femur head (56 ppm).

- Birth rates (per 1000 population) were significantly lower in B-deficient regions (15.85) compared to those in B-adequate regions (19.66) in USA.
- A study on post-menopausal women, housed in a metabolic unit, revealed that low B diet (0.25 mg/2000 Kcal) caused increased excretion of Ca and Mg and reduced serum levels of Ca ions and 17ß estradiol.
- Another study on 15 subjects (5 men, 9 post-menopausal women out of which 5 were on estrogen therapy and 1 pre-menopausal woman) fed on low Mg and marginal Cu diet, showed that B depletion (0.23 mg/2000 kcal diet) lead to low plasma Ca^{2+} and serum 25 hydroxy cholecalciferol and high serum calcitonin and osteocalcin levels. Brain function/ alertness was also affected in B-deficient subjects.

METABOLISM [59,118,209]

Absorption

Oral absorption is rapid and almost complete (approx. 99%).

Distribution and Metabolism

There is little retention but this meager amount is widely distributed with more accumulation in skeleton. Principal site of action appears to be in bones.

Excretion

Most of the absorbed B is excreted via urine. Other routes of excretion are feces and hair.

INTAKE/REQUIREMENTS [133-135,209]

	B mg/day
Daily intake from food and water	: 1.5-3.0

As essentiality of B is not established, RDA values have not been worked out. Tentative values show a wide range viz 1-13 mg/day. Humans should consume diets that supply at least 0.5 mg B/day.

MEDICINAL USES

(*a*) Boric acid is antiseptic, 3% solution is very effective for the treatment of deep wounds. The element helps healing through release of proteoglycans facilitating adhesion mechanisms. Earlier use of boric acid solution (prepared in warm water) for washing eyes has largely been replaced by better medicines.

(*b*) It is claimed to be therapeutically useful in arthritis. Newnham[131,132] claimed that about 25,000 arthritic patients were treated with approximately 70,000 bottles of a B containing formulation over a period of 3 years. The formulation, administered as tablets orally, contained borax and Mg, with some herbal ingredients and vitamins. Majority (90%) of these patients showed symptomatic relief. Shah and Vohora[161] demonstrated synergistic activity of sodium tetraborate with garlic oil in rats. The anti-arthritic effects of B have not been confirmed (or refuted) by other reports.

(*c*) Boron nucleus shows high neutron capture in cross section. Taking advantage of this fact, if B can be directed preferentially to certain cells (*e.g.*, tumour cells), it may have good potential in cancer therapy. Some organoborate compounds are reported to have such activity.[200,206]

TOXICITY [77,209]

- Boron is an industrial pollutant from coal burning. Occupational exposure in boric acid factories or general exposure of populations at places with high B content in groundwater are other sources of B toxicity.
- Borates are non-toxic but boranes are toxic. Serious poisoning occurs following ingestion of boric acid in following doses: Neonates : 1-3 g, Infants : 5 g, Adults : 20 g.
- Low oral toxicity. Chronic toxicity in experimental and farm animals (rat, dog, pig, cow) is manifested by disturbances in Ca metabolism, reduced parathyroid function and osteoporosis.
- Adverse effects on male reproductive function (decreased libido, oligospermia and infertility) have been reported.

BROMINE (Br)

CATEGORY [158]

- Possibly essential trace element.
- All metals with atomic numbers between 23 to 34 are believed to be essential. Bromine (Br), with an atomic number 35, is the next element to this critical range.
- It can replace Cl^- in the growth medium of several species of hydrophytic algae and can substitute partly the chloride requirements of chicks. While it showed stimulatory effect on growth and reproduction in chicks, 0.5 ppm bromide supplementation elicited no such action in rats.

DISTRIBUTION IN ECOSYSTEM [118]

	Br µg/g Mean (Range)
Soil	26.0 (<17.0-44.8)

HUMAN BODY [93,158,209]

Whole Body Content

Content in average adult man (60 kg): approx. 200 mg

Distribution

- Distributed in > 44 tissues and body fluids (mainly extracellular)
- Blood — 3-6 mg/litre
- Tissues — Mean 2.9 ppm (range, 1 to 9 ppm)
  Liver, 1-2 mg/kg

ROLE

- Precise role is not known.
- Can substitute I in thyroid; bromothyronine is as active as thyroid hormone.
- Serum Br levels were found to be significantly lower in uremic patients (1.10 ± 0.52 mg/l) vs. healthy controls (6.4 ± 1.7 mg/l).

DEFICIENCY

There is no known deficiency syndrome for Br.

INTAKE/REQUIREMENTS

Intake (median percentile) : 4 mg/day.[209] Requirements : not worked out.

MEDICINAL USES [77,102,195]

- Bromides exert a sedative effect. These were used earlier in cases of cough, epilepsy but now better drugs are available.
- Bromopheniramine maleate is antihistaminic, bromodiolone is anticoagulant.
- Bromobenzine has been used in Se toxicity but its efficacy is doubtful.
- Bromocriptine is used in Parkinson's disease.
- Radioactive isotope (^{82}Br) has been used for the treatment of cancers of thyroid, lungs, bladder etc.
- Local application of bromo-benzene to mouse skin inhibits and sometimes prevents the carcinogenic action of 3,4-benzopyrene.

TOXICITY [200]

- Br is less toxic vs. F and Cl
- Bromides may cause
  (*a*) Acne, skin eruptions, erythema, rashes.
  (*b*) Behavioural effects, dementia, delirium, incoordination, hallucinations etc.
  (*c*) Intracranial hypertension
  (*d*) Teratogenic effects

CADMIUM (Cd)

CATEGORY

Non-essential accumulative element. Also described as biostimulant.[59]

DISTRIBUTION IN ECOSYSTEM [15,118]

AIR

	Cd ng/m³
Remote Areas (Greenland)	0.003-1.10
North America/Europe	20
WHO guideline value (one year exposure)	10-20

North India (Ludhiana, Chandigarh)	330-21,000 (> 16-1000 times the values in USA/Europe)

WATER

	Cd µg/kg
River water	0.02
Sea water	0.10

A survey revealed Cd levels in groundwater at Delhi to be marginally above the specified Indian standards.[49]

SOIL

Surface soil (Concentration)	**Cd mg/kg**
Range (mean)	0.01-1.1 (0.5)

PLANTS [15,118]

	Bioaccumulation Index
Plant : Soil ratio	1:10
Concentration at which no sensitivity develops in immature plants	5-30 mg/kg dry matter

PLANT FOODS [12,50,118]

	Cd mg/kg (fresh weight)
Cereals (wheat, rice, rye)	0.02-0.075
Potatoes	0.03-0.05
Vegetables (lettuce, cabbage, celery, tomatoes, spinach, cucumber)	0.04-0.67
Fruits (peaches, bananas, apples, citrus fruits)	0.008-0.11
Mushrooms	0.46
Tea	0.21
Coffee	0.017

For uncontaminated foodstuffs and water, Cd is not a significant problem. Mushrooms and grains may, however, contain high concentrations. Freshwater Cd content is 100 μg/m^3 and uncontaminated foodstuffs contain < 50 μg/kg Cd wet weight. Wheat and rice grown in contaminated soil and water may, however, acquire toxic Cd concentrations.

ANIMAL FOODS [15,50,92,118]

	Cd μg/kg
Milk (considerable variation in reported range)	0.21-37
Meat, chicken	< 5 fresh weight
Higher conc. in organ meats (liver, kidney) and oyesters	200 fresh weight

MICROORGANISMS

Biomethylating organism	*Pseudomonas*

HUMAN BODY [93,118,210,211]

Whole Body Content

- Content in average adult person (mg):

Non-smokers	15
Smokers	30

- 0.7 ppm
- Placenta and mammary glands act as barriers to Cd transport into the fetus and so concentrations in newborn are extremely small. The content increases with age.

Organs

- Brain, heart, lungs, skin, liver and kidney concentrations : < 50-80 μg/g of ash.
- Wide geographical variations are reported for renal Cd content (7-fold difference between maximum and minimum values). Higher kidney Cd is observed in hypertensive subjects.

ROLE/ESSENTIALITY [209]

- No known essential function and so its presence in any cell is regarded undesirable.
- Some researchers consider this metal to have a biostimulant function. Growth stimulation (8%) was reported following increased dietary Cd (from 12.5 to 50-100 μg/kg) in rats or Cd supplementation in drinking water (16-30 μg/day) in rats.

DEFICIENCY [209]

- Some evidence of growth restriction in normal and pregnant goats is available when Cd was restricted in feed to levels < 20 μg/kg (normal: 250 μg/kg). The data could not be statistically validated.
- Human Cd deficiency syndrome is not known.

METABOLISM [15,93,118,209]

Absorption

(*a*) ***Oral***

Absorption of ingested Cd is very poor (approx. 5%). It chiefly takes place in the duodenum and ileum through passive diffusion. Uptake of Cd is inversely proportional to the Ca status of the body *i.e.*, it is strongly inhibited by Ca uptake. Increased absorption has been reported in Ca, Fe and protein deficiency states.

(*b*) ***Inhalation***

The pattern and extent of deposition of inhaled Cd depends on particulate size as follows:

Particle diameter	Part of respiratory tract
10-20 μm	nose, pharynx
5-10 μm	tracheo-bronchial region
< 5 μm	alveolar region

Distribution/Metabolism

- Distributed in > 40 human tissues and body fluids. The blood brain barrier is crossed and low concentrations of Cd reach brain. Placenta, however, is an effective barrier.
- Bound to blood cells, albumin with prolonged accumulation in tissues (half life: >20 years). Complexes in blood/plasma : cystinate, hydroxy cystinate, albumin, and aquo-Cd. Albumin prevents formation of low molecular weight complexes.
- Mostly bound to metallothionein (MT) in tissues. The metal regulates mRNAs specific for MT (50% of the total body burden occurs in liver and kidneys).
- Reacts with many macromolecules/ organic compounds of biological importance : purines, pyramidines, nucleotides, nucleosides, RNA, DNA, enzymes.
- Competes with Zn to inhibit SH-containing enzymes.
- Metallothionein (with one-third cysteine as amino acid residues) is indiffusible and protective against interaction with macromolecules of physiological importance. There is, however, a lag period of 3-4 h for metallothionein biosynthesis. During this period, binding may occur with subcellular organelles and cytosolic proteins.

SELECTED BIOCHEMICAL/ENZYMATIC EFFECTS [174]

Inhibition

(*i*) content and activity of hepatic drug metabolizing enzymes
(*ii*) protein synthesis
(*iii*) DNA synthesis *in vitro* (opposite effect *in vivo*)
(*iv*) cAMP metabolism *in vitro*
(*v*) catalase
(*vi*) carbonic anhydrase
(*vii*) phosphatases
(*viii*) vitamin-D metabolism
(*ix*) phagocytic activity of macrophages
(*x*) insulin secretion
(*xi*) nutritional elements : Ca, P, Mg, Cu, Zn etc.

Stimulation

(*i*) aldolase
(*ii*) phosphorylase
(*iii*) pyruvate carboxylase
(*iv*) fructose 6-diphosphatase
(*v*) lipid peroxidation (by inhibition of protective enzymes: glutathione proxidase and catalase)s

Excretion

Bulk of the excretion (80%) occurs through bile and feces and only a small fraction (20%) is excreted in urine. The Cd+MT complex undergoes glomerular filtration but is almost completely reabsorbed. When tubular reabsorption is impaired, increased urinary excretion may occur. The metal is retained in kidney.

INTAKE/REQUIREMENTS [209]

- Dietary intake (WHO values)

Adults	10-60 μg/day
Children	5-20 μg/day

- Maximum tolerable weekly intake: 7 μg/kg
- Normally low Cd content in most food crops (< 0.15 μg/g). Soil distribution of urban waste/sludges may significantly raise these values.

- Cereals and vegetables account for 50% of dietary intake (children : 2-25 μg/day, adults: 10-50 μg/day).
- Drinking water may contribute substantially (approx. 14%) to daily dietary intake.
- Each stick of cigarette contains approx. 1-μg Cd. Inhalatory absorption of Cd may be higher in smokers by 10-40%. It is estimated that approx. 1 mg/year is added to the body burden when a person is smoking one packet of cigarettes per day.
- There are no known requirements for Cd in the body.

GUIDELINE VALUES [208]

Drinking water (WHO)	3 μg/l
Tolerable intake (FAO/WHO)*	30 μg/day

* According to a recent report[156], this needs revision because Cd intakes well within this level also resulted in toxic effects *e.g.*, renal dysfunction and decrease in bone mineral density.

MEDICINAL USES

Cadmium sulphide (1% suspension) is used in the treatment of seborrhoeic dermatitis. It is not absorbed from the skin and systemic toxicity has not been reported from its topical use. Occasionally contact dermatitis may, however, develop.[194]

TOXICITY

Sources of Exposure/Contamination [15,118]

Due to its corrosion-resistant properties, Cd is widely used in industry. Occupational exposure may occur at the following industries:

(*a*) Smelters/metal-fuming plants
(*b*) Electroplating
(*c*) Storage batteries
(*d*) Electronic and optical equipment
(*e*) Alloys used for telephone/telegraph wiress
(*f*) Photoelectrical devices
(*g*) Stabilizers
(*h*) Solar cells
(*i*) Paints/pigments
(*j*) Nuclear reactors etc.

Some household uses *e.g.*, leaching from glazed pottery, solders in water pipes, vending machines etc. may also cause Cd contamination of drinking water and food particularly when fluids of acidic pH come in contact with these materials. Diet is the main source of Cd exposure, less than 5% of the total Cd uptake can be attributed to inhalation. Occupational exposure risk via this route, however, is high and it causes lung damage.[111]

ITAI ITAI DISEASE[15,118]

(Ouch Ouch Disease)

Disease due to overexposure to Cd reported from Toyoma region of Japan. It is characterized by short breath, choking fits, fever, headache, emphycema severe glomerular and tubular renal damage with proteinuria, bone decalcification, osteomalacia, osteoporosis, vulnerability to fractures, pain in the back and legs, and an early death. Elderly women (particularly post-menopausal) are prone to this disease. In a case study, as many as, 72 fractures were reported. Investigations traced the cause to the intake of Cd^{2+}laden water either by drinking it or by eating rice-crop irrigated with this water. The contaminated water was discharged into a river by a Zn-mining company. Exposure to Cd may not be the sole etiological factor for *itai-itai* disease. Malnutrition and vitamin D deficiency are considered to be other contributing factors.

SYSTEMIC EFFECTS [13,15,74,118,156,159,179,200,203,209]

1. ***Liver:*** Preferential accumulation occurs in liver. The hepatic content of Cd is negligible at birth and gradually increases with age. Binding occurs with metallothionein in this organ. The metal causes : (*a*) Extensive peri-portal, inter-lobular fibrosis, (*b*) Biliary hyperplasia, (*c*) Inhibition of drug metabolizing enzymes (decrease in content and activity) and (*d*) Functional liver damage: Estimation of hepatic and renal Cd concentrations, using neutron activation analyses (NAA), have been suggested to assess the degree of exposure. Protein (particularly cysteine)-rich diet protects the liver from Cd-mediated damage.
2. ***Kidney:*** Kidney is the critical organ for Cd toxicity; long-term exposure primarily affects the proximal renal tubules. The concentration of Cd is higher in the cortical region vs. that in the medulla. The complex diffuses through glomerular membrane into the tubular fluid and is almost completely absorbed at the proximal part of the tubules. The metal causes glomerular and tubular damage. This is manifested by increased urinary excretion of low molecular weight proteins which is a characteristic feature of Cd intoxication. Presence of the protein in urine ($ß_2$-microglobulin and a more stable retinal-binding protein) are of diagnostic value. These differ electrophoretically from the proteins excreted in poisoning from other metals. Other clinical features ares: (*a*) Enhanced urinary Cd excretion, (*b*) Mild/moderate histopathological changes, (*c*) Altered absorption/metabolism/ excretion of Ca, P, glucose and amino acids, and (*d*) Demineralization of bones.
3. ***Nervous system:*** Cadmium is neurotoxic and it adversely affects axonal transport. The metal crosses blood brain barrier but the concentrations in brain are relatively low vs. other organs. Symptoms include dizziness, headache, cramps and loss of consciousness. Learning disability in children is associated with elevated hair Cd concentrations.

4. ***Cardiovascular system:*** Hypertensive patients exhibit high Cd levels. In a study covering 28 American cities, death rates from all types of heart disease (except rheumatic heart disease) were significantly linked to the Cd content of urban air. Experimental hypertension has been induced by injecting Cd compounds in laboratory animals: rats, rabbits and dogs. While the precise mechanism involved in Cd-induced hypertension is not known, the possibilities include increased: (*a*) vascular resistance, (*b*) sodium retention, (*c*) renin-angiotensin activity and (*d*) vascular ineffectiveness of Atriopeptin II. Cadmium hypertensive rabbits were shown to have high Cd concentration in heart tissue. The effect on BP is produced at doses insufficient to elicit other forms of Cd toxicity. Due to interaction of Cd with Fe, decreased Fe absorption and low hemoglobin levels are observed in Cd exposed persons.

5. ***Respiratory system:*** Inhalation of Cd may cause metal fume fever which may be fatal in cases with oedema. Occupational exposure to Cd dust and fumes produces flu-like toxicity syndrome: dry sore throat, cough, severe chest pain, marked dysponea, pneumonitis and pulmonary oedema. Death may occur from generalized lung damage. Air concentrations as low as 0.1 mg Cd/m^3 may cause toxic manifestations and level > 1 mg Cd/m^3 may be fatal. Chronic exposures may lead to rhinitis, dryness and ulceration of nasal passages, loss of olfactory function, bronchitis, cough and emphycaema depending on the magnitude and duration of exposure.

6. ***Reproductive system:*** Males are reported to have higher Cd content vs. females. While this may be partly attributed to more smoking habit in males, studies in animal models revealed a true sexual dimorphism. Further estrogen is reported to facilitate fecal Cd excretion. The metal exerts effect on sex hormones and reproductive function. These include ovicidal and anti-implantation effects in females and testicular damage and reduced sperm count in males. Intra-testicular injection of Cd chloride (1-2 mg/kg) in one testicle, causes irreversible damage to the other testicle also. The metal was shown to cause marked inhibition of succino-oxidase activity and reduction Zn content of dorsolateral prostate. These properties have been used to induce sterility in stray animals: bulls and dogs. The metals Cd and Zn antagonize the effect of each other when co-administered. Human studies, however, did not reveal significant differences in blood Cd and Zn concentrations of fertile and infertile men.

7. ***Skeletal system:*** Persons with high urinary Cd excretion are reported to have low bone mineral density and more risk for fractures.

8. ***Immune functions:*** The effects resemble those of As: stimulation at low doses and inhibition at high doses.

Low dose effect:

Increase in:

(*i*) Antibody-forming cells

(*ii*) T-cell proliferation in response to mitogens

(*iii*) Response of Bcells to mitogenic challenge

Decrease in:

(*iv*) Suppressor cells (selective action)

High dose effect:

Decrease in:

(*i*) DNA synthesis

(*ii*) Primary and secondary immune response

(*iii*) Antibody titre against infection

(*iv*) Delayed hypersensitivity skin reactions

(*v*) Macrophage/PMN leucocyte activity.

The overall effect is immunosuppression leading to increased susceptibility of animals to infections and cancer induction. Tissue culture studies revealed selectively high uptake of Cd (upto 3000 times the concentration in surrounding medium) by human lymphocytes. While the precise reason for such selective and high uptake is not clear, it may have obvious immunotoxic implications for man.

9. ***Skin:*** Contact dermatitis may develop after exposure of Cd compounds.

10. ***Carcinogenic effect:*** The element is considered a human carcinogen. Studies on links of Cd exposure to the incidence of various types of cancer, showed a direct relation for lung cancer, conflicting findings for stomach cancer and no relation for prostatic cancer. Lung cancer due to Cd inhalation alone has recently been questioned. Oral uptake of Cd does not lead to tumour induction but its inhalation causes cancer. About 1 $\mu g/m^3$ Cd in the air inhaled corresponds to about 60 μg/g of the metal in lungs and it leads to 50% incidence of pulmonary tumours. The body burden and risk of cancer of Cd is considerably increased by smoking (Cd content: upto 100 ng per cigarette). Selenium and zinc have been reported to elicit protective effects against Cd-induced carcinogenesis.

11. ***Teratogenic effects:*** Injection of Cd compounds (in high doses) has been shown to induce teratogenic effects in rodents. While newborns of industrially-exposed women were underweight, no birth defects (except a few cases of rickets) were discernible in these infants.

MECHANISMS OF TOXICITY [15,50,74]

(*a*) Displacement of Zn from critical site in Zn-containing enzymes.

(*b*) Reaction with proteins and other biological molecules. High affinity for sulphydryl and imidazole nitrogen groups.

(*c*) Interference with tubular resorption of low molecular weight proteins.

(*d*) Non-metallothionein Cd and nuclear Cd are determinants of Cd toxicity. Liberation of Cd from a metallothionein-bound metal through digestion by lysosomes results in toxic effects.

(*e*) Binding of Cd to inner-mitochondrial membrane of hepatocytes causes collapse of membrane potential, depolarization and cell death.

(*f*) Inhibition of enzymes of the citric acid cycle or the respiratory chain.

(*g*) Inhibition of glucose-6-phosphate dehydrogenase activity of RBCs.

DIAGNOSTIC FEATURES

(*a*) **Characteristic symptoms:** Short breath, choking fits (ouch ouch), emphycema, demineralization of bones, osteomalacia, osteoporosis, frequent fractures, rheumatic/ myalgic pain, renal dysfunction etc.

(*b*) **Laboratory findings:** (*i*) Non-metallothionein Cd, nuclear Cd. (*ii*) Proteinuria : excretion of low molecular weight proteins in urine. $ß_2$ microglobulin provides a sensitive index for Cd toxicity. Aminoaciduria (> 200 μg/g), (*iii*) Glycoseuria.

TREATMENT [15,50]

(*a*) **Chelation therapy:** It should be quickly initiated. Delayed treatment is not effective because later the metal gets redistributed to remote sites from where it is difficult to dislodge it. Chelation can be done by agents like $CaNa_2$ EDTA (75 mg/kg/day in 6 divided doses; total dose during 5-day course should not exceed 500 mg/kg). Some agents may get harmfully redistributed to kidneys. While caution is needed in this respect for $CaNa_2$ EDTA, dimercaprol should not be used in cases of Cd toxicity as it will enhance nephrotoxicity. The preferred chelating agent is $CaNa_2$ DTPA. Unithiol may also be used.

(*b*) **Supportive measures:** Symptomatic treatment using steroids, pulmonary ventilation and respiratory support. High protein diet with adequate Ca, Zn, PO_4 and vitamin D content in diet reduces toxicity.

CALCIUM (Ca)

CATEGORY

Essential bulk element

DISTRIBUTION IN ECOSYSTEMS[118]

	Ca μg/g Mean (Range)
Soil	0.72 (0.15-0.97)

HUMAN BODY [14,93,158,210,211]

Whole Body Content

- 3.1 million atoms per billion atoms
- 1.5-2.0% of body weight
- 22.4 g/kg of fat-free tissues

- 14,000 ppm
- Total content in average adult man (60 kg): 1.0-1.5 kg

Distribution

- Presence reported in >53 tissues and body fluids
- Bones and Teeth : 99%
- Soft tissues and body fluids : 1%

ROLE 115,158,182,200,209

1. **Bones and Teeth**
   - As a constituent of bones, it provides basic structure and shape to the body and helps in movements.
   - In teeth : mastication
2. **Soft tissues and body fluids**

2.1 Regulatory function (calmodulin)

(*a*) *Enzymes*

- Phosphorylase
- Adenylate cyclose
- Glycogen synthetase
- Phospholipase
- Ca^{2+}/Mg^{2+} ATP-ase
- Pyruvic carboxylase
- Pyruvic kinase
- Pyruvic dehydrogenase
- Cyclic nucleotide phosphodiestrase etc.

(*b*) *Hormones*

- Partharmone
- ACTH : Adrenal glands
- LH : Ovaries
- cAMP : Leydig cells of testes

(*c*) *Inorganic elements*

If the levels of K, Mg, Na are high, Ca plays a corrective role. It affects bioavailability of Cu and Zn and retention of Cd, F and Pb.

2.2 Functional integrity of nervous system

2.3 Contractile mechanism of muscle tissue

2.4 Maintenance of heart beat

2.5 Blood clotting

2.6 Transport of ions across the membranes

2.7 Radiation protection: Liberal intake of Ca reduces deposition of radioactive ^{90}Sr in the body.

2.8 Geographical association: Low Ca content in water (soft water) is associated with high incidence of heart disease.

2.9 Catecholamine release

2.10 Low Ca in body fluids interferes with response to nerve stimulation. Elevated serum/CSF Ca levels have been reported in cases of epilepsy and schizophrenia.

Bones serve as homeostatic mechanism to maintain adequate Ca in blood regardless of dietary intake.

Bones → Blood and Soft tissues ←

2.11 Ca/Vitamin D may help preserve insulin-sensitivity by presenting secondary hyper-parathyroidism.

DEFICIENCY

- Children - Rickets
  - Stunted growth
- Adults - Osteomalacia
  - Osteoporosis
  - Convulsions/Coma/Death
- Laboratory tests
  - Low serum Ca
  - X ray : osteopenia

INTAKE/REQUIREMENTS

Iintake

- 320-920 mg/day[209]
- 210-1650 (median : 760) mg/day

  Highest intakes are reported in countries with 'Western' style diet rich in dairy products.[140]

Requirements

Parr and Iyengar[140] reviewed the RDA values prescribed by various agencies as follows:

Agency (year)	Age (years)	RDA (mg)	
		Males	**Females**
US National Research Council (1989)	0 – 0.5	400	400
	0.5 – 1.0	600	600
	1 – 10	800	800
	11 – 24	1200	1200
	25 – 50+	800	800
	Additional 400 mg during pregnancy and lactation.		
US NIH Consensus statement (1994)	0 – 0.5	400	400
	0.5 – 1.0	600	600
	1 – 5	800	800
	6 – 10	800 – 1200	800 – 1200
	11 – 24	1200 – 1500	1200 – 1500
	25 – 50	1000	1000
	50 – 65	1000	1000 or 1500
	65+	1500	1500
	Additional 200-500 mg during pregnancy and lactation.		
US National Academy of Sciences (1997)	0 – 0.5	210	210
	0.5 – 1.0	270	270
	1 – 3	500	500
	4 – 8	800	800
	9 – 18	1300	1300
	19 – 50	1000	1000
	51+	1200	1200
	No additional requirements specified for pregnancy and lactation.		
US Committee on Medical Aspects of Food Policy (1991)	0 – 1	525	525
	1 – 3	350	350
	4 – 6	450	450
	7 – 10	550	550
	11 – 18	1000	800
	19 – 51+	700	700
	Additional 550 mg during lactation.		

EUROPE : ILSI (1990)	20 – 59	600	800
European Communities : Scientific Committee for Food (1993)	0.5 – 3.0 4 – 6 7 – 10 11 – 17 18 +	400 450 550 1000 700	400 450 550 800 700
	Additional 500 mg during lactation For post-menopausal women: On estrogen therapy : 1000 mg/day Not on estrogen therapy : 1500 mg/day		

Dairy products, beans and leafy vegetables are rich sources of Ca.

TOXICITY [77]

Causes

- Excess absorption, overnutrition or rapid i.v. infusion
- Hypervitaminosis : Vitamin D
- Hyperparathyroidism
- Idiopathic

Symptoms

Coma, convulsions and death. Caustic alkaline substances *e.g.*, oxide, hydroxide and carbide of Ca (used as drain openers, oven and pipeline cleaners) produce irritant, corrosive effects.

CARBON (C)

CATEGORY

Essential bulk element, constituent of basic structure of human body.

HUMAN BODY [14,158,211]

Whole Body Content

- 94.5 million atoms per billion atoms
- 18.5% of total weight of protoplasm
- 230,000 ppm

- Total content in average adult man (60 kg) : approx. 16 kg

Distribution

Ingredient of all organic matter. Present in all tissues and body fluids.

Blood

- 2000 atoms in each molecule of hemoglobin.
- 28.8 mM as bicarbonate in whole blood.
- Bicarbonate is one of the main ions of the extracellular fluid.

MEDICINAL USES [200]

- None as such.
- Activated charcoal used as an adsorbant for poisons.
- Five precent CO_2 in O_2 is useful in cases of hypocapnea (CO_2 deficiency), CO poisoning and intractable hiccup. Carbon dioxide (CO_2) snow is used for destruction of warts, cavernous hemangiomas and chronic lupus erythematosus.
- Household usage in aerated drinks.
- ^{14}C is used as a diagnostic and research tool *e.g.*, for insulin clearance studies.
- Carbon monoxide (CO) is used for determining total circulating hemoglobin and lung diffusion capacity.

CERIUM (Ce)

CATEGORY

Non-essential accumulative ultra-trace element

DISTRIBUTION IN ECOSYSTEMS [118]

	Ce ppm
Earth's crust	60.0
Soil	52.3

ROLE AND TOXICITY [118]

Cerium has no nutritional role. It may replace Ca in a number of Ca-mediated biological processes affecting cAMP-dependent processes, the neuron activity, secretion of hormones, transmitters, detoxification mechanisms including calcification effects and inhibition or stimulation of enzyme activities. Gastrointestinal absorption is poor but substantial inhalatory and dermal absorption may occur. It has low toxicity. Among the lanthanide series of elements Ce citrate is least toxic and chloride most toxic (Ce Cl_3 is cystotoxic; LC: 29 mmol/L). Repeated oral intake of Ce chloride produced hematological alterations in rabbits. Intravenous injection of Ce nitrate was shown to be highly toxic in female rats. Chronic inhalatory exposure may cause pneumoconiosis in occupational setting. Elevated plasma and synovial fluid Ce concentrations have been reported in cases of rheumatoid arthritis.

CESIUM (Cs)

CATEGORY

Non-essential accumulative trace element.

HUMAN BODY [93,209]

Widely distributed, presence reported in more than 25 tissues and body fluids including all vital organs, blood, milk, skin, hair and urine.

INTAKE/REQUIREMENTS [209]

Median/percentile intake (WHO) 8.8 μg/day

As it is a non-essential element, there are no known requirements for Cs.

GUIDELINE VALUES [15,118]

Occupational exposure limit (CsOH gas) 2mg/m^3

Radioactivity guideline for drinking water

Gross beta activity for ^{137}Cs should not exceed 1 Bq/l. If this is crossed, it should be considered as a signal to investigate the cause of such increase and take remedial measures.

TOXICITY [121]

Military uses and accidental release of radionucleides may lead to contamination with radioactivity in large areas *e.g.*, by acute and protracted use of ^{137}Cs which is relatively more volatile and soluble fission product vs. U and its decay products.

CHLORINE (Cl)

CATEGORY

Essential bulk element.

DISTRIBUTION IN ECOSYSTEMS [118]

	Cl μg/g/ Mean (Range)
Soil	340 (150-623)

HUMAN BODY [14,93,158,195,210,211]

Whole Body Content

- 260,000 atoms per billion atoms
- 0.15% of body weight
- 0.2% of total weight of protoplasm
- 54 mEq/kg of fat-free tissues
- 1200 ppm
- Total content in average adult man (60 kg) : approx. 100 g

Distribution

- Widely distributed in almost all tissues and body fluids
- Presence reported in >43 tissues and body fluids.
- Major anion in extracellular fluid, less than 15% in cells.
- Significant sex differences reported for exchangeable Cl content in the body, more in females vs. males.

ROLE [79,195]

- In combination with Na, it has a role in fluid and electrolyte balance.
- Osmotic equilibrium
- Maintenance of pH
- Provides HCl for gastric juice in stomach
- Enzyme activator
- Chloride shift in bicarbonate transfer in RBCs
- Serum/CSF values show increase in nephritis and congestive heart failure and decrease in Addison's disease, diabetes mellitus, pneumonia and fevers. Urinary excretion is increased in Addison's disease and decreased in starvation and many pathological conditions *e.g.*, vomiting, pneumonia, ascites, pleuritic effusions, nephritis and heart failure.

DEFICIENCY [195]

Causes

- Dietary deficiency is unlikely.
- Conditioned Cl deficiency may occur in illness with fluid loss:
  - Diarrhoea, dysentry
  - Excessive vomiting
  - Dehydration
  - Renal disease
  - Diuretic therapy
  - Profuse sweating
  - Infants on salt-free diet

Symptoms

Anorexia, apathy, alkalosis, muscular cramps etc.

INTAKE/REQUIREMENTS [209]

Drinking water (typical concentration : 20 mg/l, maximum conc. 179 mg/l, WHO guideline value 250 mg/l) contributes upto 6% to dietary intake. Dietary intake is of little significance except in dehydratating illness.

Adequate and safe dietary intake is as follows:

	Cl mg/day
Infants upto 6 months	275-700
6 months to 1 year	400-1200
Children 1 to 3 years:	500-1500
4 to 6 years:	700-2100
7 to 10 years:	925-2775
> 11 years	1400- 4200
Adults	1700-5100

The major source for supplementation is table salt (NaCl).

MEDICINAL USES [195, 200]

- Parenteral nutrition : iv saline, dextrose saline, Na, K or NH_4 salts are used.
- Germicidal at extremely low concentrations (0.0002% Cl) used for water purification.

TOXICITY [200]

Exposure to high concentrations of Cl may cause contact urticaria. Workers handling Cl are prone to chlor acne. The lesions occur on exposed parts of the body and less frequently on the covered areas through contamination of clothes.

CHROMIUM (Cr)

CATEGORY

- Possibly essential ultra trace element
- As late as 1971, Williams[212] stated that though this element is abundant in Earth's surface, it is not found *in vivo* because it is strongly held in minerals, so unable to enter plants, food chain and then in animals and human body. Later not only its presence was detected in body, some essential functions were also discovered for this element.

DISTRIBUTION IN ECOSYSTEM [15, 49, 111, 118, 208, 209]

AIR

	Cr ng/m^3
Remote areas (Greenland)	0.6-0.8
North America	60
Europe	25
North India	11-194

WATER

	Cr µg/kg
River water	1.0
Sea water	0.2

Groundwater: Cr may get mobilized into ground water under acidic conditions. Consumption and use of such water should be restricted to protect public health.

SOIL

Surface soil	**Cr µg/kg**
Mean:	60
Range	20-100

PLANTS [15,118,147]

Critical concentration	**Cr mg/kg dry matter**
Range	5-30
Food plants	
	Cr mg/kg fresh weight
Cereals	0.1-0.4
Potatoes	0.05-0.3
Vegetables	0.11
Fruits	0.07
Mushrooms	0.06-0.13
Tea	0.95
Coffee	0.03

Unrefined beet, cane sugar, and tea are rich in Cr content. Bloniarz and coworkers[34] examined selected herbs, herbal fruit teas and their infusions for Cr content. The amounts present were found to be quite safe for human health.

ANIMAL FOODS [15,118]

	Cr per kg fresh weight
Milk and milk products	10-60 µg
Meat/Pork/Beef	0.1-30 mg
Eggs	1.91 mg
Liver/Kidney	0.2-0.4 mg
Sea foods	0.05-0.07 mg
Sea fish	0.02-2.0 mg

Oyesters are rich in Cr content

HUMAN BODY [15,93,158,210,211]

Whole Body Content

- 0.6×10^{20} atoms in the body
- 6×10^{5} atoms in each cell
- 0.09 ppm
- Content in average adult man (60 kg) : approx. 1.4 to 5.0 mg

Distribution

- Distribution in > 45 tissues and body fluids including all vital organs. Crosses blood-brain and placental barriers.
- Blood – Serum : 2-20 μg/L
  – RBCs : 37 (19-66) μg/L
- Tissue Cr content is 10-100 times its blood levels.
- High concentration in nuclear proteins/RNA.
- Hair content is a good index for nutritional status of Cr.

ROLE/ESSENTIALITY [10,50,59,115,120,148,209]

- Trivalent Cr is considered to be an essential element but this has recently been questioned. Cr is needed for the biosynthesis of glucose tolerance factor (GTF); lack of this factor causes diabetes type II. There is considerable experimental evidence for its essentiality and probable role in carbohydrate metabolism and diabetes mellitus. Evidence in human beings, at the present state of knowledge, is indirect and incomplete. Tissue Cr concentrations decrease with age.
- Cr supplements enhance the metabolic action of insulin and lower the risk factors of cardiovascular disease.

DEFICIENCY [78,79,120,209]

Animal Models

Experimental deficiency is reported to cause impaired glucose tolerance, growth, and longevity, diabetes, cataract and atherosclerosis in animal models. The response of isolated liver mitochondria to insulin is decreased in these animals. These symptoms are reversed by dietary supplementation with chromium chloride.

Human Beings

- Dietary deficiency is not known.
- Marginal deficiency may occur in certain situations. Patients on total parenteral nutrition have lower serum/urine Cr levels than normal people. High carbohydrate diets causes excess urinary Cr excretion and predisposes to deficiency.
- Abnormal Cr metabolism is reported in multiparous insulin-dependent diabetic women.
- Diabetic patients have 33% less Cr vs normal healthy subjects. Toe nail Cr analysis revealed lower Cr content in diabetics and CVD patients vs healthy controls. Besides low levels diabetics show poor Cr utilization.

METABOLISM [118,209]

Absorption

- It depends on the ionic form; trivalent form (Cr^{3+}) is poorly absorbed (< 1%), hexavalent (Cr^{6+}) form is better absorbed (2-6%).
- Primary site of gastro-intestinal absorption is jejunum.
- Absorption in juvenile and insulin-dependent diabetic patients is 2-4 times higher vs healthy subjects.
- Higher absorption occurs when the Cr is linked to amino acids and other biomolecules.
- Absorption also occurs through skin and inhalatory route. The latter is of special importance for occupational exposure in many industries. Persons employed in leather tanning industry and construction workers are prone to substantial cutaneous absorption.

Binding/Metabolism

- Diffusion occurs across plasma membrane in the form of organic complexes following binding. This is necessary for distribution to various tissues and body fluids.
- Hexavalent Cr^{6+} is reduced to Cr^{3+}. The latter gets bound to ß-globulin fraction of serum proteins especially transferrin and also to hemoglobin.
- Reduction of Cr^{6+} following entry into cell membranes makes it immunologically active and less toxic.
- Normally transferrin is only 30% saturated with Fe. Chromium (Cr^{3+}) has affinity for transferrin. It competes with Fe^{2+} for the same sites. Therefore patients of hemochromatosis (with >50% Fe saturation) retain less Cr is normal or Fe-depleted (anaemic) subjects. These patients are less prone to Cr toxicity.

Excretion

- Excretion is mainly renal. It is biphasic. Initial phase is rapid which clears the element from blood. Second phase is slow; it removes Cr from tissues.
- Marginal excretion occurs through bile, feces, hair, and sweat.
- Higher excretion is reported in (a) diabetic patients and (b) following oral glucose load in healthy subjects.

MEDICINAL USES [79,195,200]

- In study on 12 malnourished children (6 each from Jorden and Nigeria), administration of Cr Cl_2 250 µg restored glucose tolerance test to normal.
- Improvement of glucose tolerance (50-60%) was observed in maturity onset diabetic patients of all ages.

- Hyperglycaemia controlled in patients on prolonged total parenteral nutrition.
- In an Indian study administration of 5 drops of 0.05 M $CrSO_4$ twice daily was reported to elicit nervine tonic action. This is an isolated report; no other study is available to confirm or refute these claims.

According to a recent report,[116] Cr picolinate exerts a rapid and favourable impact on glycemic control in patients with corticosteroid-induced diabetes. Ample intake of bioactive Cr may have the potential to reverse the negative influence of corticosteroids on insulin signaling. Such an effect might have utility not only for smokers but also for other subjects in whom chronic upregulation of the hypothalamic-pituitary adrenal axis compromises vascular health. Supplements of Cr (alongwith Mg and antioxidants) have been used in complimentary therapies for diabetes mellitus without adverse effects. The evidence for their routine use is, however, insufficient. Long-term risk/benefit assessment studies are warranted for such usage.[72]

INTAKE/REQUIREMENTS [118,209]

- Estimated intake through food, water, and air

USA	:	110 µg/day
India	:	150 µg/day

- Recommended Dietary Allowance (Tentative):
  50 - 200 µg/day

GUIDELINE VALUES [111,118,208]

- Drinking water **Cr µg/l**

Permissible (WHO)	:	50
Excessive (India)	:	50

- Occupational exposure limit

(OEL in air on 40h work week) Cr^{6+}Hexavalent Cr	:	0.05 mg/m^3
Other forms of Cr	:	0.5 mg/m^3

- Biological exposure limit in urine : 15 µg/g of creatinine
- Listed by EP under hazardous waste category

TOXICITY [6,15,50,77,96,98,111,114,118,197,209]

Trivalent Cr has low toxicity, hexavalent Cr is highly toxic.

Lipid Peroxidation

- Cr enhances lipid peroxidation.
  - Cr^{3+} forms complexes with lipophilic ligands which diffuse into cells easily.
  - Cr^{6+} penetrates membranes and oxidizes protective SH groups to disulphide bridges. This form is more toxic.
- Main toxic effects on skin and respiratory system.

Sources of Exposure/Contamination

From industrial and personal uses of Cr alloy in:

(*a*) Stainless steel
(*b*) Chrome plating
(*c*) Dyes/Pigments
(*d*) Leather tanning
(*e*) Textiles
(*f*) Cassette tapes
(*g*) Magnetic storage media for computers
(*h*) Pyrotechnics
(*i*) Photography
(*j*) Welding plants
(*k*) Seed disinfection
(*l*) Construction work (as impurity in cement) etc.

SYSTEMIC EFFECTS

1. ***Liver:*** Following ingestion or inhalation, it accumulates in liver causing damage with cirrhosis, enlargement and dysfunction of this organ. In patients of hepatic disorders, blood Cr levels are reported to be lower vs healthy subjects.
2. ***Kidney:*** It causes renal tubular damage similar to that observed in cases of Hg poisoning. Rats given a subcutaneous injection of 10 mg potassium dichromate showed symptoms of oligouria, proteinuria and glycoseuria with histological changes and decreased enzymatic activity. Regeneration occurred after three weeks.
3. ***Cardiovascular system:*** Chromium has a role in cholesterol homeostasis. When rats were given Cr in drinking water (1-5 mg/ml), serum cholesterol levels and stainable lipids in aorta decreased but hepatic fatty acid synthesis was increased. Patients of atherosclerosis show less Cr excretion in urine vs. healthy individuals. Toxic exposure to chromates causes methemoglobinemia.

4. ***Skin:*** Chromates are corrosive and allergenic in nature and cause contact dermatitis, eczema and slow healing ulcers. Some of the lesions become lepromatous but a direct association with this disease has not been proved. Occupational exposure in construction/tanning industry workers may cause chronic contact dermatitis.

5. ***Respiratory system:*** Exposure causes allergenic and inflammatory symptoms in the respiratory tract. Perforation of the nasal septum, bronchial asthma and lung cancer may also occur.

6. ***Reproductive system:*** Chromium was shown to induce reproductive impairment in female rats. An increase in estrogenic activity and decrease in androgenic and myotrophic effects of testosterone propionate has been reported with this element. With advancing pregnancy urinary Cr excretion increases but hair Cr content is proportionately decreased.

7. ***Immune function:*** The metal acts as a hapten which conjugates with proteins and causes immunotoxic effects affecting cellular and humoral immunity and non-specific host-defence mechanisms. Experimental studies revealed inhibition of (*i*) T-dependent antibody response, (*ii*) ß-lymphocyte proliferation, (*iii*) Lymphokine production, (*iv*) Phagocytic activity and (*v*) Chemotaxis. Clinically skin reactions and asthmatic bronchitis are attributed to effects on immune function.

8. ***Carcinogenicity:*** Hexavalent Cr easily penetrates cell membrane and enters the cell. It reacts with H_2O_2 to produce reactive oxygen species. Occupational exposure has been associated with high risk for cancers of nasal septum, lungs and skin. Effluents from textile/dye industries of Sanganer district of Jaipur (Rajasthan, India) showed high mutagenic activity. Chromium is highly clastogenic (human cells more sensitive vs rodent cells to chromosomal damage). Cytogenic studies on chromate workers revealed increase in sister chromatid exchange and chromosomal aberrations in peripheral hepatocytes. On parenteral administration, the findings regarding its carcinogenicity were inconclusive. Scalp hair of patients with breast cancer revealed significantly higher content vs healthy subjects.

9. ***Teratogenicity:*** Both trivalent and hexavalent Cr compounds induced teratogenic effects in experimental animals : mice, chicks and golden hamster. No such effects were recorded in human beings inspite of higher Cr concentrations (%) in placental (Non exposed : 3 µg, Exposed : 13.5 µg) and fetuses (Non exposed : 9.28 µg, Exposed : 114 µg).

MECHANISMS OF TOXICITY [15,118,184]

- Corrosive, Allergenic nature
- Dermal membranous absorption of immunologically active forms.
- Oxidative stress, enhancement of lipid peroxidation, DNA damage; inhibition of DNA-polymerase by free radicals.
- Carcinogenic action.

TREATMENT [15,118]

- Removal of contaminated clothing
- Washing of skin with water, dressings soaked in EDTA
- Chelation therapy : Unithiol
- Monitor hepatic and renal function
- Symptomatic treatment

COBALT (Co)

CATEGORY

Essential ultra trace element.

DISTRIBUTION IN ECOSYSTEM [15,118]

AIR	**Co ng/m^3**
Remote areas (Greenland)	0.001-0.90
Rural areas	1.0-28
USA	0.2-83
Europe	0.4-18.3
WATER	**Co mg/m^3**
Sea water	0.02
Fresh water	0.20
Drinking water limits	Not available
SOIL	**Co mg/kg**
Average concentration in surface soil	8

PLANTS [118]

Critical concentration at which sensitivity develops in immature plants	15-50 mg/kg, dry weight
Plant Foods	**Co mg/kg, fresh weight**
Cereals, vegetables, fruits, tea, coffee	0.02-1.00

ANIMALS

	Co ppm
Average whole body content in wild animals	0.2-0.5

Foods of animal origin are good sources of Co.

HUMAN BODY [14,158,200,209-211]

Whole Body Content

- 5 atoms per billion atoms
- 450,000 atoms in each cell.
- 0.03 ppm
- 0.021 mg/kg of fat free tissues
- Total content in average adult man (60 kg) : 1.5 - 3.0 mg

Blood	**Co μg/L**
Whole blood	0.30-0.99
Tissues	**Co μg/g ash**
Brain, Heart, Kidneys, Liver, Lungs etc.	< 2-17

Distribution

- Widely distributed in more than 43 tissues and body fluids.
- Constituent of cobalamine (Vitamin B_{12}) which contains 4.35% Co. Also present in inorganic form.

ROLE/ESSENTIALITY [50,200]

(*a*) As Vitamin B_{12}, it blocks some enzymes involved in Fe transport. This induces intracellular hypoxia and stimulates RBC formation.

(*b*) Cyanocobalamin is essential for normal functioning of all cells including nerve cells.

(*c*) The role of inorganic Co present in tissues and body fluids is not precisely known.

DEFICIENCY [118,200]

- Primary deficiency is rare except in strict vegetarians. Deficiency states may occur due to:

  (*a*) Lack of gastric intrinsic factor

  (*b*) Gastrectomy

  (*c*) Malabsorption syndromes

- Vitamin B_{12} deficiency causes **Pernicious anaemia** mostly in elderly persons. It is manifested by:
  (*a*) Decreased RBC count and hemoglobin level
  (*b*) Numbness in limbs
  (*c*) Short breath/Fainting
  (*d*) Pallor
  (*e*) Diarrhoea
  (*f*) Fever
- The deficiency syndrome rarely occurs in persons below 30 years in age as chronic megaloblastic anaemia. It is manifested by macrocytic (but not hyperchromic) erythrocytes with elevated colour index and is usually associated with lack of gastric intrinsic factor.
- The deficiency syndrome responds to treatment with:
  (*a*) Liver extract
  (*b*) Vitamin B_{12}

METABOLISM [118,209]

Absorption

A substantial part (63-93%) of orally-ingested Co is absorbed. Absorption also takes place through inhalation and skin. These are reported to be the main routes of its occupational exposure. Absorption of Co is influenced by Fe status. Anaemic patients absorb more Co. Absorption antagonism is reported with Fe, Mg and Mn.

Distribution/Metabolism

While Co is widely distributed in the body, the principal sites of storage are liver, spleen, kidneys (prolonged retention), endocrine glands, lymph nodes and bones. Interactions occur with many trace elements particularly Fe and enzymes.

Excretion

Excretion occurs through feces (60-80%) and urine (20-30%). It is biphasic, the first 24-hour excretion is very fast followed by a slow phase. Most of the excretion (90%) is complete within 8-10 days. Microquantities are excreted slowly in sweat, saliva, seminal fluid, hair and nails. Inhaled Co is rapidly cleared via exhaled air.

INTAKE/REQUIREMENTS [118,209]

	Co µg/day
Median dietary intake (range)	15 (6.2-43.0)
Estimated requirements	3-5

Generally the requirements are met by normal diet.

GUIDELINE VALUES [118,209]

	Co µg/m^3
Occupational Exposure Limit	50-100
(Air concentrations on 40-h work week)	
Biological Exposure Limit	Co µg/L
Blood	0.65-1.27
Urine	0.50-1.70

MEDICINAL USES [127,137,153,195]

Co is used as Vitamin B_{12} for the treatment of Pernicious anaemia and not as metal as such. Co alloys are used in orthodontics and ^{60}Co for radiotherapy in cancer patients. The effect of gama knife thalamotomy (GKT) was studied in Parkinson's disease-related tremor after reloading of Co. In the majority (80-85%) of cases treated after reloading, tremor and rigidity showed substantial reduction around 6 months after GKT. Cases treated before reloading showed the two lesion types in both series (restricted and defuse). After reloading, the lesion volume was reduced. The shorter delay in clinical improvement and smaller lesion size were attributed to the increased radiation dose. Gama knife radiosurgery is a patient-friendly procedure. It has expanded internationally with over 170 sites worldwide treating over 250,000 patients. It uses focused beam of ^{60}Co radiation.

TOXICITY [15,118]

Sources of Exposure

From industrial/personal uses in:

(*a*) Glass
(*b*) Ceramics
(*c*) Paints
(*d*) Varnish
(*e*) Resins
(*f*) Alloys in tooth prosthesis
(*g*) Cyanocobalamine in medicine

SYSTEMIC EFFECTS [15,50,200,209]

1. ***Hemopoietic system:*** Excess of Co causes **Polycythemia** with increase in globular elements of the blood and stimulation of RBC production (erythrocytosis). Large amounts of $CoCl_2$ were, however, reported to depress RBC production. A goitre like syndrome has also been reported. Accidental intoxication in children is manifested by cyanosis, coma and death.

2. ***Liver:*** Experimental studies revealed rapid fluxes of Co between this organ and rest of the body. Hepatic concentrations of Vitamin B_{12} show decrease and those in serum are increased in various diseases *e.g.*, cirrhosis, viral hepatitis.
3. ***Kidney:*** Co chloride has been used for induction of experimental nephrotoxicity in rabbits.
4. ***Nervous system/Beer drinkers disease:*** Co is added in beer to stabilize froth. Excess consumption of beer may damage eighth cranial nerve causing deafness, coma and death. Co gelatin has been used to induce focal epilepsy in rats.
5. ***Cardiovascular system:*** Cardiomyopathy occurs in Beer drinker's disease. It is manifested by short breath, ECG changes, cyanosis and heart failure. Myocardial degeneration is observed on autopsy. Both experimental and human studies are available for such effects.
6. ***Respiratory system:*** Occupational exposure to Co containing dusts may cause respiratory irritation, pneumoconiasis, pulmonary fibrosis and chronic lung disease with symptoms of dyspnoea and olfactory dysfunction.
7. ***Skin:*** Co chloride (1% solution) has been shown to cause cutaneous sensitivity in women. It has been included among the European battery of 24 patch tests for contact dermatitis.
8. ***Reproductive system:*** Co nitrate is reported to protect testes from Cd-induced damage. Deficiency is associated with reduced fertility.
9. ***Immune function:*** Immunosuppressive effects (against humoral immunity and host resistance using viral infection and tumours) have been demonstrated in various experimental animals.
10. ***Carcinogenicity:*** While mutagenic and carcinogenic effects have been shown in some experimental studies, there is no evidence for such effects following occupational exposure in human beings. Some reports, however, indicate higher incidence of bronchial carcinoma among Co miners.
11. ***Teratogenic effects:*** Studies with Co chloride (upto 5 mg/kg) in rats revealed reduced ossification and fetal size and also embroyotoxic effects but no fetal abnormalities. Pregnant women receiving Co chloride (75-100 mg/day) for the treatment of anaemia showed no fetal malformations.

MECHANISM OF TOXICITY [15,47,118]

- Decreased oxidation of pyruvate in heart muscle causes myocardial toxicity.
- Skin sensitization is mediated through immune mechanisms.
- Inhibitory effect on cytochrome P_{450}, transferrin and heme synthesis in large doses.
- Potential to produce active oxygen species and interference with DNA repair system.

TREATMENT

- Chelation therapy with Di-sodium calcium EDTA i.v. or Dimercaprol i.m.
- Antihistaminics and other symptomatic measures.

- Vitexina (a product containing Vitexin derived from a medicine plant (*Vigna radiata*) was recently shown to elicit radioprotective effects in breast cancer patients undergoing ^{60}C therapy.[84]

COPPER (Cu)

CATEGORY

Essential trace element.

DISTRIBUTION IN ECOSYSTEM [49,111,118]

AIR

	Cu ng/m^3
Remote Areas (Greenland)	0.029-12
North America	100
Europe	340
North India	208-2682

WATER

	Cu mg/m^3
Sea water	0.3
Fresh water	3

Groundwater: Cu may get mobilized into it from the soil under acidic conditions. Consumption and use of such water should be restricted to protect public health. The level of Cu in Delhi ground water was found to be marginally above the specified Indian standards.

SOIL

	Cu mg/kg
Mean (Range)	23 (1-80)

PLANTS [15,118]

	Cu mg/kg dry matter
Concentration at which no sensitivity develops in immature plants	20-100

Plant foods

	Food	Cu mg/kg (fresh weight)
Low 0.6-5.0 mg/kg	Cereals	2.4-5.0
	Potatoes	1.57
	Vegetable	1.00
	Fruits	0.6
	Mushrooms	4.9
High 8-22 mg/kg	Radish	8-22
	Coffee	13.3
	Tea	21.8

Recently Cu bioaccumulation in Chinese cabbage (*Brassica pekinensis* Rupr) and Cu toxicity were reported. Though the plants with elevated Cu content suffered damage to some extent as a result of Cu treatment, they looked healthy. The treatment stimulated (instead of reducing) the chlorophyll content. Lack of visible symptoms of damage poses risk to human health from the transfer of metal in food.[214]

ANIMAL FOODS [118]

	Food	Cu mg/kg fresh weight
Low 0.19-15 mg/kg	Milk and milk products	0.19-3.92
	Meat, pork, beef, chicken	1.19-7.13
	Eggs	2.44
	Fish	0.7-15
	Sea foods	3.5
High 20-190 mg/kg	Liver	50 (20-190)
	Oyesters	upto 137

HUMAN BODY [14, 36,93,118, 158, 210, 211]

Whole Body Content

- 170 atoms per billion atoms (15.3 million atoms in each cell)

- 2 mg/kg of fat-free tissues.
- Newborn : 4.7 ppm
  Adults : 1.7 ppm
- Content in average adult man (60 kg) : 75-150 mg

Distribution

- Widely distributed; reported in at least 51 tissues and body fluids.
- Blood

	Cu μg/L
Plasma (Ceruloplasmin)	1120 (610-1420)
RBC (Erythrocuperin)	980 (750-1310)

- Large amounts in brain, liver (principal organ for storage and metabolism), heart, kidneys, skin, and pigmented parts of the eye.
- Integral part of DNA/RNA molecule.
- Constituent of many enzymes.

ROLE/ESSENTIALITY 78,118,149,187,209

- Role in hemopoiesis; required for hemoglobin formation and, therefore, oxygen transport.
- Transfer of Fe from tissues to plasma requires the oxidation of ferrous to ferric form. This is catalysed by Cu.
- Role in formation of bones and aortic elastin.
- Enzymatic functions.

Constituent of the enzyme	Symptoms associated with absence or deficiency
Cytochrome oxidase	Tissue respiration blocked
Ceruloplasmin (Laccase)	Cu transport disrupted
Ascorbic acid oxidase	Disturbed redox reactions
Lysine oxidase	Cartilage formation stopped
Tyrosinase	Melanin formation affected Albinism and Leucoderma
Superoxide dismutase	Cell destruction by free radicals
Monoamine oxidase	Neurotransmitter synthesis affected

- ***Hormonal function:*** Cu salts stimulate gonadotropin releasing hormone and hence LH release.
- ***Infectious diseases:*** Serum/plasma Cu levels are elevated (with rise in Cu : Zn ratio) in most of the infectious diseases including acute viral hepatitis, thalassemia, pulmonary tuberculosis, leprosy, schistosomiasis, legionellosis etc. This is attributed to the mobilization of ionic (Cu existing in the organism) when pathogenic action begins.

DEFICIENCY [50,62,78,85,87,209]

Experimental Animals

- Deficiency in experimental animals (rats) has been reported to cause progressive thinning of aortic wall and even aortic rupture which is fatal. Lack of GnRH release in Cu-deficient rats and g.pigs cause infertility.
- Loss of 'startle response' in the offsprings of Cu-deficient mother rats.
- Sway back in lambs born to mother on Cu-deficient pastures.

Infants

- **Hypochromic, microcytic anaemia:** Generalized pallor. The symptoms respond to combined therapy with Fe and Cu. Concurrent protein deficiency may also exist.
- **Scurvy-like symptoms:** In malnourished infants rehabilitated on high calorie/low Cu diet, the following symptoms are observed: anaemia, neutropenia, neonatal ataxia, diarrhoea osteopenia and scurvy-like bone changes.
- **Menke's Kinky Hair Syndrome or Trichopoliodystrophy:** It is inherited as a X-linked recessive trait with defect in Cu transporting ATPase. It inhibits Cu absorption and is manifested by cerebral degeneration, steely hair (kinks are formed on bending), muscle hypotonous, seizures and death.
- **Occipital Horn Syndrome:** It is a rare X-linked recessive disturbance of Cu metabolism. It is characterized by marked connective tissue features *e.g.*, lax skin, loose joints, hernias, bladder diverticulae and skeletal abnormalities. Decreased activity of lysloxidase (a Cu-dependent enzyme involved in cross linking of collagen and elastin) has been proposed as the underlying mechanism for this syndrome.

Adults

- According to a recent report[62], Cu intake in UK population is rarely adequate which is a matter of concern, both in terms of public health and possible clinical consequences.
- Deficiency may occur in patients on: (*a*) prolonged total parenteral nutrition and (*b*) Zn therapy (Cu and Zn antagonize each other). The symptoms include hypercholesterolemia, lack of aortic elastin leading to thinning of aortic wall/rupture.
- Inborn error of tyrosine metabolism disrupts normal melanin formation pathway causing leucoderma or albinism.

METABOLISM [15,118,187,209]

Absorption

(*a*) ***Oral***

– Absorption from gastro-intestinal tract : 30-50%

– Mainly from duodenal mucosa through a Cu-binding protein.

– Oral absorption depends on:

Chemical form: Inorganic Cu (I), Cu (II) Organic

Copper status: Increased absorption occurs in Cu deficiency.

Diet: Presence of substances which inhibit Cu absorption include phytate, high ascorbic acid, certain amino acids and ligands which form complexes with Cu, and metals Cd, Hg, Mo, Ag, Zn etc.

(*b*) ***Inhalation:*** Absorption may occur from respiratory tract from exposure to dusts, fumes and mist.

(*c*) ***Skin***

- Absorption of Cu can take place through intact skin. Traditionally Cu bracelets are used for the treatment of muscular and cardiovascular ailments. It has been reported that upto 50 mg of Cu per month may be absorbed by the user.
- Tracer studies revealed perfusion of Cu through intact cat skin and the formation of Cu glycinate complex under aerobic conditions.
- The metal is probably oxidized by amino acids present in sweat.

DISTRIBUTION/METABOLISM [15,118]

- Binding occurs with albumin. Bound forms (Cu-albumin complex and ceruloplasmin) get transported to different tissues and body fluids.
- Liver is the key organ for storage and metabolism of Cu where its distribution is as follows:

Soluble fraction	:	52%
Nuclei	:	15%
Mitochondria	:	12.4%
Microsomes	:	14%

Excretion

Major route of excretion is through feces and bile both for unabsorbed ingested as also injected Cu. Less than 50 μg/24 h is excreted in urine and negligible amounts through sweat, hair and menstrual flow.

INTAKE/REQUIREMENTS [118,209]

Earlier reports indicated dietary intakes of approx. 5 mg/day but more recent studies using duplicate sample analysis technique suggest that actual intakes may be very low (1-1.5 mg/day) and with 30-50% oral absorption, these may not meet the recommended dietary allowances (RDA) which are 2-3 mg/day.

GUIDELINE VALUES [118,209]

Occupational exposure limit (OEL) in ambient air for 40 h work week	0.1-1.0 mg/m^3
Biological exposure limit for hepatic Cu	250 µg/g dry weight
Maximum permissible concentration in agricultural soil	100 ppm or 2-3 mg/kg/ hectare/year
Drinking water (India)	
Permissible	1 mg/l
Excessive	3 mg/l

MEDICINAL USES [79,141,195,200]

- Insecticides, fungicides, pesticides
- Intra-uterine contraceptive devices (IUCDs)
- Complexes with anti-inflammatory drugs (nifumic acid and phenylbutazone) are reported to enhance their activity.
- Copper bracelets are used traditionally with claimed value in arthritis and cardiovascular diseases.
- Capsules containing copper chloride 1-3 mg per day po or 200 µg i.v. given twice a week have been reported to elicit clinical benefit in cases of leucoderma. Though the precise etiology of this disease is not known, it has been attributed to an inborn error of metabolism/defect in melanin synthesis which involves tyrosinase, a copper containing enzyme. Clinical utility in this disease has not been proved without doubt.
- Acute diarrhea: use in combination with Zn.

TOXICITY

Sources of Exposure/Contamination [15,198]

From extensive uses as Cu *per se* or in the form of alloys (brass) in:

(*a*) Kitchenware

(*b*) Water pipes/taps

(c) Electrical goods
(d) Pigments
(e) Algicide/fungicide/rodenticide preparations
(f) IUCD
(g) Supplements in deficient pastures etc.

Acute human poisoning may occur from:

(a) Accidental/suicidal ingestion of gram quantities of soluble salts specially copper sulphate.
(b) Topical application of Cu preparations on extensive burns/eroded skin
(c) Hemodialysis

Grape Garden Sprayer's Disease [15,42,118,198]

Toxicity may result from occupational exposure to herbicide sprays (Bordeux mixture which contains $CuSO_4$ and lime) in vineyard workers. The disease affects both lung and liver. Hepatosplenomegaly, blue lungs (due to Cu deposits), granulomas and portal stenosis are the prominent symptoms. It may also occur through inhalatory exposure to dust, fumes and mist at work place. Periodic estimations of serum alkaline phosphatase level (which is elevated) has been recommended for identifying workers prone to hepatic damage from occupational exposure.

Indian Childhood Cirrhosis [50,155,198]

This disease is reported in children ingesting Cu in milk or water boiled/stored in brass/copper utensils. Higher incidence recorded in certain communities in Rajasthan. Tin coating of utensils prevents release of Cu in milk/water and so is protective against ICC.

Schizophrenia [185,200]

It is believed that excess tissue Cu can cause this disease. This has, however, never been proved or refuted with authentic research data. The patients of schizophrenia show high serum and low CSF levels of Cu. This is consistent with the hypothesis of reduced activity of Cu-dependent enzymes in schizophrenia.

Wilson's Disease (Hepatolenticular Degeneration) [50,155,196]

This disease is caused by a rare autosomal recessively inherited defect characterized by impaired incorporation of Cu in ceruloplasmin and inhibited biliary Cu excretion. This results in accumulation of Cu in many organs including liver, brain, kidneys and eyes. The symptoms include hepatic dysfunction, yellow atrophy of liver, cirrhosis, hemochromatosis, anaemia, spasticity, rigidity, treamours, behavioural/personality changes, aggressive outbursts low serum ceruloplasmin, high hepatic Cu levels and urinary Cu excretion. The neurological manifestations of the disease may not be observed in many cases.

SYSTEMIC EFFECTS [15,42,77,195,197,199,200,209]

1. ***Liver:*** Excess oral intake of Cu causes liver damage and may even lead to fatal hepatitis. Elevated Cu and Cu-bound protein levels are observed in varied hepatic ailments both in adults and children. These include neonatal hepatitis, Indian childhood cirrhosis, alcoholic hepatitis, primary biliary cirrhosis, intra- and extra-hepatic biliary atresia, hemochromatosis, fatty liver, neoplasms, Wilson's disease etc. Because of wide variations in reported baseline values, hepatic Cu estimations are not of much significance or diagnostic value in most cases. Exceptions include prolonged choleostasis, chronic biliary cirrhosis and Wilson's disease (with values upto 30 times the control levels) where such estimations are useful. Elevated serum Cu concentrations have been reported in acute viral hepatitis, ICC, Laennec's cirrhosis, choleostasis, chronic active hepatitis, obstructive and hemolytic jaundice, alcohol withdrawal syndrome (with hallucinations and delirium tremens), and malignancy. The practical utility of such estimations remains to be worked out.
2. ***Kidney:*** Renal damage occurs following exposure to excess Cu. Rats receiving $CuCl_2$ injections (1-4 mg/kg for 236 days) exhibited degeneration and sloughing of epithelial cells of the proximal convoluted tubules. These cells contained yellow droplets which showed positive histochemical reaction for Cu. The other parts of nephron were unaffected. Elevated renal Cu accumulation occurs in Wilson's disease and high urinary Cu excretion (upto 1500 μg/day, normal : 215.2/μg/day) is observed in this disease and also as a non-dialyzable complex in nephrosis. There is concurrent increased elimination of Fe, Zn and some proteins bound to these metals. High serum Cu levels have been reported in cases of uremia and renal failure.
3. ***Nervous system:*** Toxic accumulation of Cu occurs in brain in cases of Wilson's disease (Please see page 79). The neuropsychiatric manifestations of this disease include spasticity, rigidity, treamours, wild choreform movements and schizophrenia. High serum/plasma Cu concentrations are observed in schizophrenia and mentally-retarded patients practicing pica.
4. ***Cardiovascular system:*** The cardiovascular symptoms of Cu toxicity, include tachycardia, hypotension, hemolysis, hemolytic anaemia, methemoglobinemia hematuria cardiovascular collapses and death. Elevated serum/plasma Cu levels have been reported in some cardiovascular diseases *e.g.*, atherosclerosis, congestive heart disease (CHD) and rheumatic heart failure. The metal is present in myocardium, forms an integral part of DNA/RNA molecule and blood (ceruloplasmin in plasma and erythrocuperin in RBCs). An imbalance of Cu and Zn metabolism probably contributes to increased risk of CHD. Breast milk, with optimum Zn: Cu ratio, is therefore better vs. cow milk. Breast feeding is associated with less incidence of cardiovascular diseases. Patients undergoing hemodialysis may introduce sufficient Cu into patients's circulation to cause hemolysis.
5. ***Respiratory system:*** Inhalatory exposure to Cu dust/fumes/mist at work place may lead to nasal congestion, perforation of nasal septum, pulmonary Cu deposition and fibrosis. Abnormally high serum Cu levels are observed in chronic infectious and malignant diseases *e.g.*, tuberculosis and bronchial carcinoma (Please also see under Grape garden sprayer's disease, page 79).

6. *Skin :* Leucoderma and albinism are caused by an inborn error of metabolism involving tyrosinase (a Cu containing enzyme). The normal pathway for melanin synthesis is disrupted leading to patchy or generalized lack of skin pigment. Elevated serum ceruloplasmin concentrations are observed in many skin diseases including lepromatous leprosy. Copper compounds possess antiseptic, germicidal and fungicidal properties and are used in topical skin preparations.

7. *Reproductive system:* Copper salts stimulate gonadotropin releasing hormone and LH release producing ovulation. These salts are, therefore, used for experimental induction of ovulation in laboratory animals. A study on the cervical mucus of 17 regularly menstruating women revealed significantly lower Cu values in ovulatory and post-ovulatory phases vs those in the pre-ovulatory phase. Addition of Cu ions to ovulatory mucus alters its rheological properties making it unfavourable for sperm penetration. This property is the basis for the use of Cu in IUCD. Serum Cu levels rise with progress of pregnancy. After second trimester, a slight decline is noted but the values tend to rise again towards the onset of labour and marked elevation has been reported at term. Infertile women exhibit lower serum Cu levels vs fertile women. Oral contraceptives have also been shown to induce alterations in serum Cu.

   The metal has been shown to depress androgenic and myotrophic effects of testosterone and reduce % of motile sperms *in vitro*. A comparative study on 80 infertile and 88 men of known fertility revealed higher plasma Cu concentrations in the former but no differences were discernible for their seminal plasma Cu levels. Some reports for lower Cu values in oligospermic and azoospermic men are also available.

8. *Immune function:* Adverse effects are observed on immune function by both deficiency and excess of Cu. Experimental deficiency was shown to impair both cellular and humoral immune responses in rodents. Exposure lead to reduction in T cell dependent antibody response in mice and chemotaxis in rabbits.

9. *Carcinogenic effect:* Cu (II) is known to cause depurination of DNA, an event which may lead to mutagenesis. Experimental induction of cutaneous cancer (mice) and testicular teratoma (fowl) using $CuSO_4$ has been reported. Cutaneous application of carcinogen results in epidermal loss of Cu. Biochemical studies reveal significantly higher Cu concentrations in serum/plasma of patients with various types of cancer e.g. carcinomas (bronchi and breast), sarcoma/osteosarcoma, leukemias and Hodgkin's disease. Occupational exposure is associated with a higher incidence of lung cancer in coppersmiths.

10. *Teratogenic effect:* While experimental evidence exists for Cu-induced teratogenicity in hamsters, no human reports for such effects are available.

MECHANISM OF TOXICITY [15,118,209]

(*a*) Local irritation of gastric mucosa.

(*b*) Impaired lysosomal excretion of hepatic Cu in bile.

(*c*) Hepatic accumulation and excretion of Cu in bile in Wilson's disease is due to a genetic defect in Cu excretion.

(*d*) Enhanced lipid peroxidation SH-groups oxidized to disulphide bridges, formation of stable complexes with glutathione, reduced availability of antioxidants, oxidation of catechols by tyrosinase of semiquinone free radicals.

(*e*) Release of hepatic Cu into blood and extracellular fluids causes damage to susceptible cells specially those of brain and liver.

DIAGNOSTIC FEATURES [15,118,209]

History

History of accidental or suicidal ingestion or occupational exposure.

Clinical presentation

Characteristic symptoms of gastrointestinal irritation (salivation, epigastric pain, nausea vomiting, diarrhoea) alongwith intravascular hemolysis, jaundice, tachycardia, hypotension, passage of blood elements in urine, fatal cardiovascular collapse or renal failure. Detection of Kayser-Fleischer ring in occular cornia is diagnostic for Wilson's disease.

Laboratory investigations

Elevated hepatic Cu concentrations (> 250 μg/g dry matter) and low plasma ceruloplasmin levels (< 20 mg/dl) are diagnostic for Wilson's disease. Hepatic Cu estimations may also be of diagnostic value in prolonged choleostasis and chronic biliary cirrhosis as the values in these diseases may be upto 30 times higher vs those of healthy controls.

TREATMENT [15,118,209]

Chelation therapy

D-penicillamine is drug of choice in cases of acute poisoning and Wilson's disease. A total dose of 0.5 to 2.0 g po per day may be administered in divided doses preferably 1-2 h after meals to avoid chelation of dietary metals. While this agent is specific for Cu and can be given orally, it can not be given in persons allergic to penicillin. Alternative chelating agents have to be used in such cases. Other chelating agents used include Na_2 Ca EDTA, Dimercaprol, Trientine, DMPS and Unithol. Dimercaprol (300 mg i.m. per day for 10 days) has been successfully used as an adjuvant to D-penicillamine in cases of Cu poisoning and Wilson's disease. Trientine (Adults: 0.75-1.0 g/day, children: 0.5-1.5 g/day) has orphan drug status for Wilson's disease and so is given when D-penicillamine is not tolerated.

Other measures

- Oral Zn acetate and ammonium tetrathiomolybdate (25-50 mg three times a day) may help reduce toxicity by decreasing Cu absorption and its uptake by hepatocytes.

- Exchange transfusions with albumin-enriched peritoneal dialysis.
- Hepatic grafts: If the graft survives, Cu metabolism may be normalized and the patient may become symptom free. Hazards of immunosuppression need to be closely monitored.

DYSPROSEUM (Dy)

CATEGORY

Non-essential accumulative ultra-trace element.

DISTRIBUTION IN ECOSYSTEM [118]

Earth's crust	3 ppm

HUMAN BODY [93,193]

Presence has been detected in whole blood, serum, lungs, lymph nodes, prostate glands and tooth enamel.

TOXICITY [118]

Oral absorption is poor but significant absorption may take place from inhalatory and dermal routes. It has low toxicity. Mice fed Dy oxides, continuously over 3 generations, exhibited no differences in mortality, morbidity, morphological development, growth rate and reproduction capacity between the treated and control groups.

ERBIUM (Er)

CATEGORY

Non-essential accumulative ultra-trace element.

DISTRIBUTION IN ECOSYSTEM [118]

Earth's crust	2.8 ppm

HUMAN BODY [93,193]

Presence has been reported in whole blood, serum, lungs, and tooth enamel.

ROLE AND TOXICITY [118]

Erbium interacts with actin, prevents tubule formation and causes alterations in enzyme activities.

EUROPIUM (Eu)

CATEGORY

Non-essential accumulative ultra-trace element.

DISTRIBUTION IN ECOSYSTEM [118]

Earth's crust	1.2 ppm

HUMAN BODY [93,193]

Presence has been detected in whole blood, serum, lungs, lymph nodes and tooth enamel.

TOXICITY [118]

Low toxicity. Mice fed Eu oxide over 3 generations, showed no ill-effects on growth rate, reproduction, morphological development or survival time.

FLUORINE (F)

CATEGORY

Essential trace element

DISTRIBUTION IN ECOSYSTEM [209]

AIR

Industrial fumes and dusts from chemical or smelting plants may significantly contribute to environmental fluoride.

WATER

Natural waters (content shows wide variations)	< 0.1 to > 20 mg/l
USA, Central Europe	low content vs Asian and many African countries

HUMAN BODY [14,93,158,210,211]

Whole Body Content

- 125 atoms per billion atoms
- 37 ppm
- Total content in average adult man (60 kg): approx. 800 mg

Distribution

- Presence reported in > 25 tissues and body fluids
- Mineralized tissues : 99% (Bones : 1000-5000 ppm).
  Soft tissues : 1% (2-5 ppm)

ROLE [118,209]

- Needed for optimum health of bones and teeth.
- Growth (?)

DEFICIENCY [51,112,118,143,209]

- Dental caries
- In areas where fluoride content in water is low, fluoridation (1 ppm) reduces the incidence of dental caries.
- Growth retardation reported in rats on low dietary intake of F

INTAKE/REQUIREMENT [209]

	Total intake in adults	0.2-2 mg
	Intake from breast milk in 3 month-old infants (6-country study)	3-74 μg
	Safe intake levels depend on age, upper limits are as follows :	
Infants	1 year	0.5 mg
	2 years	1.0 mg
	3 years	1.5 mg
Adults		5.0 mg

METABOLISM [180,209]

Absorption

From drinking water	> 90%
From diet	30-60%

Absorption mainly takes place from upper intestines. Significant absorption has been reported from fluorinated toothpastes in children.

Distribution/Metabolism

Mainly retained in teeth and bones

Excretion

Approximately 80% of the absorbed F is excreted in urine daily. Also secreted in milk.

MEDICINAL USES

Dental Caries: some recent reports describe at length the issues involved in identifying, protecting and restoring childrens oral health,[51] successes and drawbacks in caries-preventive use of fluorides,[112] and the WHO approach for the prevention of dental caries in the 21st Century.[143]

TOXICITY [73,118,180,209]

- Corrosive and toxic effects.
- Froldfalics can cause vegetative and material damage (specially in particulate form). It is readily taken up by plant leaves. Extremes of pH and leachibility of ionic species enhances the damage.
- *Fluorosis* occurs when fluoride content in water is > 8 ppm. About 62 million people in India in 16 out of the 32 states are affected with dental, skeletal and non-skeletal forms of fluorosis.
  - Mottling of teeth. Weak dental enamel
  - Increased bone density. Knock knee
  - Radiological features : osteosclerosis, osteoporosis, osteomalacia
  - Neurological disturbances
  - Renal damage
  - Lung damage may also occur
  - Endemic genu valgum in India, Kenya, Tanzania
- ***Acute poisoning*** may occur by accidental ingestion of insecticides/ rodenticides.
  - Colic, nausea, vomiting
  - Hypocalcaemia
  - Nervous irritability
  - Respiratory paralysis. Death

  Ingestion of large amounts of F (5-40 mg/day) in drinking water produces severe skeletal deformity.

- ***Biochemical Mechanisms***
  - Mg depletion
  - Inhibition of Mg-dependent enzymes
  - Decrease in cell ATP level
- ***Genotoxic Effects***

  Controversial findings and opinions. A recent report[150] found no relationship between sub-chronic fluoride intake and DNA damage in Wistar rats.
- ***Fatal Dose of NaF***

  Adults : 5 g

  Children : 0.5 g
- ***Treatment***
  - Gastric lavage
  - Intravenous glucose or Ca gluconate
- ***Fluoride in Tooth Paste***

  Indiscriminate addition should not be permitted as it can be used by subjects in areas with excess F in water with harmful effects.

  A recent review[54] critically discussed the health risk assessment approach to have a quantitative look at fluorosis, fluoride exposure and intake in children.

FRANCIUM (Fr)

CATEGORY

Not reported in human body.

GADOLINIUM (Gd)

CATEGORY

Non-essential accumulative ultra-trace element.

DISTRIBUTION IN ECOSYSTEM [118]

Earth's crust	5.4 ppm

HUMAN BODY [93,118,193]

Presence has been reported in whole blood, serum, lungs, lymph nodes, skeletal muscles, and tooth enamel.

TOXICITY [118]

Experimental sarcomas were produced in mice using Gd compounds.

GALLIUM (Ga)

CATEGORY

Non-essential accumulative element

DISTRIBUTION IN ECOSYSTEM [118, 158]

AIR

Values not available. Exposure to biosphere is increasing with greater use in semiconductors.

WATER

Sea water	0.03 ppb

SOIL

Content in Earth's crust	5×10^{-4} %

PLANTS

Wide variations in different species	10 ppb to 2 ppm dry matter

ANIMALS

Mammalian muscle	1.4 ppb
Bovine liver	5-8 ppb

Marine fish have very high content of Ga

HUMAN BODY [93]

Whole Body Content

Not available

Distribution

Presence reported in at least 24 human tissues and body fluids.

Blood	< 80 μg/L
Tissues	**Ga μg/g**
Brain	12.80
Heart	810
Kidney	15.50
Liver	15.70
Lungs	0.05
Spleen	2930
Testes	0.002

ROLE/ESSENTIALITY

Ga has an atomic number 31 which falls within the critical range 23-34 of essentiality but, at the present state of knowledge, it has no biological function.

DEFICIENCY

There is no known deficiency syndrome for Ga both in animals and man. Pulmonary exposure to Ga oxide and arsenide leads to substantial absorption (36-44%).

METABOLISM [118]

Absorption

Gastrointestinal absorption of Ga is very poor. It is not enhanced by Fe deficiency.

Distribution/Metabolism

Distribution is wide. Retention in body is influenced by renal function. Binding occurs with siderophores, lactoferrin and transferrin. Distribution is influenced by inflammation and malignancy.

Excretion

Studies on experimental animals, indicate that excretion occurs mainly through urine following oral intake and through fecal route on pulmonary exposure. Excretion is quite rapid.

INTAKE/REQUIREMENTS

Dietary intake values are not available and RDA has not been worked out as Ga is a non-essential element.

GUIDELINE VALUES

Not available

MEDICINAL USES [50,94]

It is used as a chemotherapeutic and radio-imaging agent. Because of its cytotoxic properties, Ga nitrate has found therapeutic applications in the treatment of some tumours. Experimental studies suggest its potential utility in sarcomas and carcinomas including adenosarcoma, fibrosarcoma, leukemia, lymphoma and Hodgkin's disease. Radioactive ^{67}Ga has been used for diagnostic and monitoring purposes in inflammatory and infectious disease. For tracer studies it is used in citrate form in ng concentrations.

TOXICITY [50]

Sources of Exposure

Increasing use of Ga compounds, particularly Ga arsenide, in superfast integrated circuits for semiconductors and telecommunication operations, emissions in biosphere will rise and may pose a threat to environment. Other uses are in electronic industry, optics, chemotherapy and radioimaging. Air pollution also occurs from burning coal and petroleum products.

Toxic Effects

Adverse effects depend on route of exposure and type of compound used (phosphide, antimonide, trimethyl/tetramethyl Ga, or arsenide). Arsenotoxicity may result from Ga As. It is volatile and so exposure at work place may be hazardous in the absence of guideline values. It is cytotoxic with principle effect on kidney. *Experimental studies* in rats and mice showed hypercalciuria, tubular necrosis and shortening of life span. Treatment with Ga As produces morphological damage to renal mitochondria and inhibits formation of cerebrospinal fluid in rats by reduced HCO_3 production. Biochemical effects include inhibition of aminolevulinic acid (ALA) in blood, liver and kidneys and glutamate dehydrogenase *in vitro*. *Human studies* also revealed nephrotoxic effects as evidenced by enhanced blood urea N values, decreased creatinine clearance rate and hypercalciuria. Anaemia was also observed in exposed subjects. Toxic effects are also exerted on liver and hemopoietic system. Inflammatory action on respiratory tract may be seen following pulmonary exposure.

MECHANISM OF TOXICITY [50]

(*a*) Local irritant/ inflammatory effects

(*b*) Cytotoxic action by alterations in metabolism of Ca, Fe and Mg.

TREATMENT

(*a*) Administration of osmotic diuretics attenuates nephrotoxicity and hypercalciuria.

(*b*) Specific antidotes are not available. So, symptomatic treatment/supportive measures are used for the management of Ga toxicity.

GERMANIUM (Ge)

CATEGORY

Possibly essential element

DISTRIBUTION IN ECOSYSTEM [118]

AIR

Not available.

WATER

Sea water	
Surface	0.0005 ppb
Depth	0.009 ppb

SOIL

Content in Earth's crust	0.0007%
Soil USA	0.6-1.3 mg/kg

PLANT FOODS [118]

Content in plants	0.1-1.0 ppm
Some medicinal plants contain higher amounts	
Wheat bran	1.23 μg/g
Tomato juice	5.76 μg/g

ANIMAL FOODS [118]

Low content in meat	
Mammalian muscle	0.14 ppm
Fish and sea food	1.2-2.3 μg/g
Milk and dairy products	1.2-1.5 μg/g

HUMAN BODY [93,158]

Whole Body Content

- < 1 ppm
- Content in average adult man (60 kg) : 20 mg

Distribution

Presence reported in at least 20 human tissues and body fluids including all vital organs *e.g.*, liver, heart, brain, kidneys, spleen, pancreas, testes.

Blood		Ge mg/L
Whole blood	:	0.44-5.00
Erythrocytes	:	0.65
Serum	:	< 0.04-0.29

Tissues		Ge µg/g
Brain	:	2.61
Kidney	:	9.00
Liver	:	0.04
Lungs	:	0.09
Testes	:	0.50
Hair	:	2.30

ROLE/ESSENTIALITY [59,118]

With an atomic number of 32, Ge falls within the critical range (23-34) of essentiality and shares many properties with Si. While no precise function is known for Ge, it affects immune function as follows:

Increase	Decrease
Interleukin-1	Antibody production (50%)
Interferon activity	
Natural killer cell activity	

DEFICIENCY

There is no known Ge-deficiency syndrome.

METABOLISM [118]

Absorption

Absorption occurs both through oral and inhalatory routes.

Distribution/Metabolism

After absorption Ge gets distributed to various tissues and body fluids. Greater retention was observed in spleen, brain and vertebrae of rats. The half life is estimated to be 1.5-5.0 days. Biotransformation occurs in liver. It involves catalysis by cytochrome P-450 system through C-hydroxylation mechanisms.

Excretion

Excretion is rapid and mainly through urine.

INTAKE/REQUIREMENTS [118]

Intake varies with type of food

	Ge µg/day
High protein, low carbohydrate diet:	400
Selected ovovegetarian diet:	3500

RDA values have not been worked out

GUIDELINE VALUES [118]

Occupational Exposure Levels (OEL)	
for inorganic-Ge compounds USSR	1-2 mg/m^3 air
Biological exposure limits	Not available

MEDICINAL USES [118,200]

(*a*) **Antitumour effects:** Ge blocks cellular proliferation at very low concentrations and suppresses protein, RNA and DNA biosynthesis and human tumour cells *in vitro*. These studies also revealed synergistic action of SGe with 5-fluorouracil and cisplatin. Because of these properties, it has been used for therapeutic effect in various types of cancers *e.g.*,

- Breast cancer
- Carcinoma of cervix
- Prostate cancer
- Renal carcinoma
- Non-Hodgkin lymphoma
- Metastic carcinoma etc.

Intravenous injection was given with a 100 ng/l solution as a bolus dose per day. The efficacy is, however, low (<20% response in breast cancer at MTD) with narrow therapeutic index (causing neurotoxic effects).

(*b*) **Analgesia:** Experimental studies in rats indicated potential of morphine analgesia. This property gives an added benefit in chemotherapy of advanced carcinomas which are associated with pain.

(*c*) **Anaemias:** Use in anaemias has now been abandoned. It is only of historical interest.

(*d*) **Antimicrobial Action:** Aryl Ge compounds have been reported to possess antibacterial and anti-viral effects *in vitro* but no *in vivo* reports are available for such effects.

TOXICITY [118,200]

Sources of exposure

Through industrial or personal uses in :

(*a*) Semiconductors

(*b*) Catalysts

(*c*) Medical imaging devices

(*d*) Dental castings with Ag-Cu-Ge alloys

(*e*) Glass for lenses used in cameras

(*f*) Anti-tumour agent

(*g*) Welding works etc.

Toxicity

Experimental studies: Ge has been shown to cause rough skin, renal failure and reduce longevity in rats.

Human studies

(*a*) Industrial exposure to fumes in welding workers causes Ge toxicity manifested by diarrhoea, dehydration, bradycardia, hypotension, and injury to lung capillaries and splanchnic areas.

(*b*) Neurotoxicity has been observed following medicinal uses. The symptoms include hypothermia, dizziness, numbness in extremities, blurred vision, impaired coordination and seizures.

(*c*) There is no evidence for carcinogenic or teratogenic effects in human beings.

MECHANISM OF TOXICITY [118]

(*a*) Cytotoxic action

(*b*) Effects on immune system

(*c*) Direct irritant effect on respiratory mucosa.

TREATMENT

Symptomatic treatment.

GOLD (Au)

CATEGORY

Non-essential accumulative element.

DISTRIBUTION IN ECOSYSTEM [118]

AIR	**Au ng/m^3**
Czechoslovakia	5.2
WATER	**Au ng/L**
Oceans	4.0
Groundwater: Au may get mobilized into it from the soil under acidic conditions. Consumptions and use of such water should be restricted to protect public health.	
SOIL	**Au µg/kg**
Earth's crust	5.0

PLANTS [118]

Some plants accumulate gold *e.g.*, Garden balsams.

HUMAN BODY [93,158,193]

Whole Body Content

- 0.1 ppm
- Content in average adult man (60 kg) : < 10 mg

Distribution

Gold is reported present in at least 39 tissues and body fluids. Half of the total body burden is in bones.

Blood	**Au µg/L**
Whole blood	0.35
Tissues	**Au µg/g ash**
Brain, heart, liver, Kidneys, lungs, skin	< 10

ROLE/ESSENTIALITY

At the present state of knowledge, Au has not been attributed with any essential function.

DEFICIENCY

No Au deficiency syndrome reported.

METABOLISM [22]

Absorption

Some phosphine containing Au complexes (*e.g.*, Auranofin) are absorbed from the gastro-intestinal tract. Absorption is poor and it is influenced by the oxidation state of Au and ligands present.

Distribution/Metabolism

After absorption, most of Au gets bound to proteins (>85% to albumin). Protein bound Au diffuses across cell membranes including that of RBCs. It concentrates in liver, kidney, synovial fluid and lysosomes. Interactions occur with cyanide (inhaled by tobacco smokers) and some anti-arthritic drugs *e.g.*, d-penicillamine. Detoxication involves reduction of Au (III) to Au (I) by SH containing proteins.

Excretion

It is excreted through feces and urine. Renal clearance is < 20% for oral Au preparations (*e.g.*, Auranofin). In contrast, it is > 60% for parenteral Au preparations (*e.g.*, Myocrisin, Solagnol).

INTAKE/REQUIREMENT

Au is a non-essential element. So, dietary intake and RDA values have not been worked out.

MEDICINAL USES [15,22,61,89,104,200]

- It has been used earlier for the treatment of many diseases, without notable success, *e.g.*, asthma, leprosy, syphilis, tuberculosis etc. These uses have now been discontinued in favour of better and specific drugs.
- Now it is used medicinally only for the treatment of **Rheumatoid Arthritis.** Chrysotherapy is associated with several problems:
  - (*a*) Not effective in all cases; 20% patients get no benefit.
  - (*b*) Low therapeutic index; 25-40% patients develop toxic reactions. These may be very severe in half of them necessitating discontinuation of therapy.
  - (*c*) High-relapse rate.
  - (*d*) Interactions with other anti-arthritic drugs.
- Curcumine gold complex, developed by Indian scientists from gold and anti-inflammatory principle of turmeric (*Curcuma longa*), is reported to be an effective drug for the treatment of arthritis.
- Calcined gold preparations *Swarna Bhasma* used in Ayurveda and *Kushta Tila Kalan* used in Unani medicine have recently been shown to exhibit immunostimulant (in contrast to

the known immunodepressant effects of Au preparations used in modern medicine), analgesic, anticataleptic, glycogen sparing/antifatigue, antioxidant, nootropic and neuroprotective actions in experimental animals with wide margin of safety.[22–26] These preparations exhibited anti-oxidant and restorative effects against global and focal models of ischemia in rats and attenuated stress-induced alterations in brain catecholamines, serotonin and plasma cortisterone levels.[162–64]

- A recent review [48] revealed interesting results with Au (I) and Au(II) compounds in cancer chemotherapy. The toxicity was, however, high.

TOXICITY [88,118,154,157,160]

Toxicity may occur from its anti-arthritic use only. No evidence is available for its toxic effect from environmental/industrial exposure. Gold is used in:

(*a*) Coinage

(*b*) Jewellery

(*c*) Electronic industry

(*d*) Dentistry

(*e*) Medicine : mainly as an anti-arthritic drug.

Gold toxicity is manifested mainly by its immunosuppressants, hemopoietic and cutaneous effects:

(*a*) Aplastic anaemia

(*b*) Thrombocytopenia

(*c*) Mucocutaneous reactions.

SYSTEMIC EFFECTS [15,39,61,82,89,104,157,200]

1. ***Liver:*** Hepatotoxic effects, including hepatoma by gold thioglucose (GTG) therapy, have been reported. It should not be used in patients with liver disease.
2. ***Kidney:*** Nephrotoxicity is a common side effect of gold therapy. So, it is not advisable to use it in patients with concurrent renal disease.
3. ***Nervous system:*** Toxic manifestations of gold therapy may include encephalitis, EEG abnormalities and peripheral neuritis.
4. ***Respiratory system:*** Inflammation of respiratory passages including pneumonia.
5. ***Skin:*** Cutaneous manifestations of Au toxicity include erythema, urticaria, rash and diffuse slate-coloured pigmentation.
6. ***Reproductive system:*** Experimental studies showed anti-ovulatory effects in rats and mice.
7. ***Immune function:*** Anti-inflammatory/antiarthritic effects of Au are due to its inhibitory action on immune function. Toxic immunosuppression is manifested by blood dyscriasis and mucocutaneous reactions. Skin reactions to Au jewellery are rare but these may be observed in patients on Au therapy.

8. ***Gastrointestinal system:*** Gastrointestinal disturbances may occur during treatment with Au compounds.

MECHANISM OF TOXICITY [15,61]

Partial or complete myelosuppression

TREATMENT [15]

(*a*) Discontinue Au therapy
(*b*) Chelation with Dimercaprol
(*c*) Symptomatic treatment including steroids (for pneumonitis) and supportive measures

HAFNIUM (Hf)

CATEGORY

Non-essential accumulative ultra-trace element.

DISTRIBUTION ECOSYSTEMS [118]

Soil	4.12 ppm

HUMAN BODY [93,193]

Presence has been detected in human blood and tooth enamel.

GUIDELINE VALUES [118]

Occupational exposure limit	0.5 mg/m^3 air

TOXICITY [118]

Hf may contribute to the local effects of fixed prosthesis/ceramic implants.

HELIUM (He)

CATEGORY

Inert gas. Not reported in human body

HOLMIUM (Ho)

CATEGORY

Non-essential accumulative ultra-trace element.

DISTRIBUTION IN ECOSYSTEM [118]

Earth's crust 1.2 ppm

HUMAN BODY [93,193]

Presence has been detected in whole blood, serum, lungs and tooth enamel.

HYDROGEN (H)

CATEGORY

Essential bulk element. Constituent of basic structure of human body.

HUMAN BODY [14,118,158]

Whole Body Content

- As water (H_2O) : 70% of the body
- 630 million atoms per billion atoms
- 9.5% of total weight of protoplasm
- 100,000 ppm
- Total content in average adult man (60 kg): approx. 7 kg

Distribution

- Ingredient of all organic matter.
- Present in all tissues and body fluids.

ROLE [158]

- Metabolic activity in living organisms leads to continuous formation of H but free H ion within most body fluids is very small and constant.
- Buffers (sodium bicarbonate, phosphates), proteins and esters limit the pH and maintain it at optimum level.

INDIUM (In)

CATEGORY

Non-essential trace element.

DISTRIBUTION IN ECOSYSTEM [118]

Present in low concentrations in the environment

AIR	**In ng/m^3**
Average concentration	0.30
High concentrations in some residential areas of Belgium	1.91
Higher concentrations near smelting works	5.79
WATER	**In ng/L**
Sea water	0.1-0.7
SOIL	
Earth's crust	10^{-5}%
Content in soils near smelter works	2.05 mg/kg

PLANTS AND ANIMALS [118]

Average In content	Below detectable limits to 10 μg/kg in beef and ham.
Marine organisms near smelter works	Upto 1.5 μg/kg

HUMAN BODY [93]

Values for total body content are not available. Presence reported in only 4 human tissues and body fluids : blood plasma (< 4 μg/L), serum (< 8 μg/L), lungs and tracheobronchial lymph nodes (0.62 μg/g). Parenteral administration of colloidal In shows accumulation in liver, kidney, and spleen.

ROLE/ESSENTIALITY

At the present state of knowledge, In is a non-essential element.

DEFICIENCY

There is no known In deficiency syndrome.

METABOLISM [50,118]

Absorption

The absorption of In from gastro-intestinal tract is very poor (< 2%). Moderate absorption occurs following inhalatory exposure.

Distribution/Metabolism

Experimental studies revealed that most of the parenterally administered In is taken up by tracheoendothelial lymph nodes. Inhalatory exposure leads to deposition in major airways with little alveolar uptake. Ionic In is transported in blood after binding with transferrin. Tissue distribution and accumulation depends on the ionic form of In. Major sites are reticuloendothelial system, liver and kidney. Binding occurs with high molecular weight cytosolic proteins.

Excretion

The excretion depends on the chemical form : ionic form is mainly excreted in urine and the colloidal In complexes mainly in feces.

INTAKE/REQUIREMENT

Not known.

GUIDELINE VALUES [118]

Not available. Some US authorities suggested maximum air levels of In as 100 ng/m^3 of air.

MEDICINAL USES [50]

(*a*) In may be used intra-venously as a diagnostic agent to localize malignant and inflammatory lesions.
(*b*) Indium oxide is used in medicine for organ scanning and treatment of liver tumours.

TOXICITY [50]

Sources of Exposure

(*a*) Used in semiconductor industry for the production of high-speed semiconductors.
(*b*) Medicinal and diagnostic uses described above.
(*c*) Used in various soldering alloys as a hardening agent.
(*d*) Poisoning from environmental/occupational exposure is rarely reported because of its low concentrations in the environment and poor absorption. Such problems may arise from local waste in future due increasing use of In-compounds in semiconductors or other high technology industries.

Symptoms

Experimental

The metal is relatively inert but salts exert toxic effects when given parenterally. Doses of 2-5 μg/kg were shown to produce liver and kidney damage in rats and dogs. Orally, soluble salts are less toxic. Reduction in life span of rats and mice has been reported following In exposure. Administration in drinking water (5 ppm) for life elicited no ill effects in mice.

Human

No reports of human toxicity are available.

Mechanism of Toxicity [50]

Precise mechanisms have not been elucidated. Biochemical and ultrastructural studies indicate damage to structure and function of endoplasmic reticulum.

IODINE (I)

CATEGORY

Essential trace element.

DISTRIBUTION IN ECOSYSTEM [118,208]

WATER	**I μg/l**
Wide range reported	2-15
Content in goiterogenic areas	0.1-2.0
SOIL	**I μg/g Mean (Range)**
Content	11.0 (7.0-16.1)

High rainfall or floods leach out Iodine from soil and all food grown in such areas are I deficient or goiterogenic. Himalayan region, mountain ranges of China, Ganga valley in India and Bangladesh are I-deficient. According to WHO, about 1600 million global population is at risk of IDD.

PLANT FOODS [118,209]

	I μg/g fresh weight
Cereals grains	47 (22-72)
Fruits	18 (10-29)
Legumes	30 (23-36)
Vegetables	29 (12-201)

ANIMAL FOODS [118,209]

	I μg/g fresh weight
Milk	47 (35-56)
Meat	50 (27-97)
Fresh water fish	30 (17-40)
Marine fish	532 (163-3180)
Cooking reduces the I content of food as follows :	
Frying	20%
Grilling	23%
Boiling	upto 58%

HUMAN BODY [14,93,158,218]

Whole Body Content

- 0.2 ppm
- Content in average adult man (60 kg) : 10-20 mg.

Distribution

Presence reported in >21 human tissues/body fluids. A major part (70-80%) of the total body burden is present in thyroid gland and 90% of the total thyroid I occurs as thyroglobulin. Intra thyroid I is reported to be elevated in persons over 60 years.

Blood		**I μg/dl**
Protein bound I in serum	:	
New born	:	7.9
Adults	:	5.4
Erythrocytes	:	Absent
Tissues		**I μg/g fresh weight**
Brain	:	0.02 ± 0.002
Liver	:	0.20 ± 0.06
Kidneys	:	0.04 ± 0.01
Lungs	:	0.07 ± 0.03

Thyroid gland: Total content 8-12 mg; I concentration in this gland is more than 100-fold higher than in any other tissue or body fluid.

Significant concentrations present in orbitary fat and orbicular muscle.

ROLE/ESSENTIALITY [118,209,218]

- Essential constituent of thyroid hormones: thyroxine and tri-idothyronine.
- Regulation of basic metabolic rate (BMR), growth and development.
- Role in reproductive function and lactation.
- Severe illness, not directly related to thyroid, affects thyroid function and I content in young and mature age persons (Age: 14 to 60 years). High intra thyroid I values have been reported in malignant tumors, cardiovascular disease, renal insufficiency, hepatic cirrhosis, pneumonia, tuberculosis, sepsis etc.

DEFICIENCY [118,209]

- Deficiency causes:
  (*a*) Cretinism
  (*b*) Goitre
  (*c*) Hypothyroidism
- Prolonged deficiency impairs reproductive function and may cause sterility.
- Effects are observed at all stages of development (physical and mental); from fetal stage to adult life. According to WHO, the term 'goitre', in use so far, now needs to be broadened to a wider designation viz. iodine-deficiency disorders (IDD) as follows:

The spectrum of Iodine Deficiency Disorders

Stage of development	**Disorder**
Fetus	Abortions Stillbirths Congenital anomalies Increased perinatal mortality Increased infant mortality Neurological cretinism (mental deficiency, deaf mutism, spastic diplegia, squint) Myxoedematous cretinism (dwarfism, mental deficiency) Psychomotor defects
Neonate	Neonatal goitre Neonatal hypothyroidism

Child and adolescent	Goitre Juvenile hypothyroidism Impaired mental function Retarded physical development
Adult	Goitre with its complications Hypothyroidism Impaired mental function Iodine-induced hyperthyroidism
All ages	Increased susceptibility to nuclear radiation

Laboratory Tests for Deficiency/Goitre

(*a*) **Serum :** Reduced thyroxine (T_3) and tri-idothyronine (T_4) levels and elevated thyroid stimulating hormone (TSH) concentrations. The latter is carried out by radioimmunoassay and is considered a preferred method particularly for pregnant women and neonates.

(*b*) **Urine :** Iodine excretion (24 h) is reduced.

METABOLISM 209

Absorption

Absorption is 100% and occurs from all parts of the gastro-intestinal tract.

Distribution/Metabolism

Through distributed in > 21 tissues and body fluids, the storage occurs principally in thyroid gland for formation of T_3 and T_4 hormones.

Excretion

Urine is the main route of excretion. Some excretion also occurs in feces, milk and sweat.

INTAKE 209

	I µg/day
Approximately dietary intake	205

Table salt (iodized) and sea food are good sources of I.

REQUIREMENTS [209]

	I μg/day
Infants upto 6 months	40
6 months to 1 year	50
Children 1-10 years	70-120
Adults	150
Additional requirements	
Pregnancy	125
Lactation	250

Intakes should be increased in presence of goiterogenic diets.

MEDICINAL USES

- Iodides are uses as:
  – Expectorants
  – Germicidal agents for external application on wounds, abrasions etc.
  Popular preparations are tincture iodine and iodine lotions/solutions. Idophores are used for similar purposes. These cause less pain but their germicidal efficacy is also less vs. that of iodides (1% in 70% ethanol).
  – Counter-irritant ointments for muscular pain.
  – Contrast media for radiographic purposes.
- Burnt sponges (with high I content) were used by ancient Greeks to treat goitre.

TOXICITY [77]

Intakes > 2 mg/day are considered excessive. Ingestion of 4 g I and 40 ml of tincture iodine are reported to be fatal.

- **Thyrotoxicosis** occurs following excess intake of iodine with symptoms of exophthalmic goitre and high urinary I excretion.
- Impairment of fertility and lactation.

- Acne
- Maternal exposure to I^{131} may be hazardous for developing thyroid gland.
- Corrosive to mucus membranes of gastro-intestinal tract, and causes pulmonary irritation (if inhaled).

TREATMENT [77]

- Goiterogenic foods
- Anti-thyroid drugs or radioiodine.
- In cases of poisoning, do not induce emesis, maintain airway, give intra-venous fluids and treat bronchospasm and edema.

IRIDIUM (Ir)

CATEGORY

Non-essential accumulative ultra-trace element.

DISTRIBUTION IN ECOSYSTEMS

Emitted from volcanoes

HUMAN BODY [93,193]

Presence has been reported in blood and tooth enamel.

IRON (Fe)

CATEGORY

Essential trace element.

DISTRIBUTION IN ECOSYSTEM [15,118]

AIR	**Fe ng/m³**
Remote Areas (Greenland)	166-171
North America	829-2000
Europe	130-5900
WATER	**Fe mg/L**
River water	0.67
Sea water	0.01 - 0.14
SOIL	**Fe mg/kg**
Content in soil	0.7 - 4.2

FOODS PLANTS [15,118]

	Fe mg/kgf
Cereals	26-46
Potatoes	8
Vegetables	14.7
Fruits	5.3
Tea	172
Coffee	168

Legumes and Spinach are rich in Fe.

ANIMAL FOODS [15,118]

Milk and milk products	0.7-1.9 mg/100 kcal, 300-400 µg/L
Meat/pork/beef/chicken	> 200 mg/100 k cal Higher concentration in organ meats, liver/kidney vs. muscles.
Shell fish	> 2 mg/kg

HUMAN BODY [93,118,158]

Whole Body Content

- 38,500 atoms per billion atoms
- 75 mg/kg of fat-free tissues
- 60 ppm
- 0.006% of body weight
- Content in average adult (60 kg): 4.2 g

Distribution

- Present in all living cells and therefore in all tissues and body fluids.

Blood

Whole blood	:	40-60 mg/100 ml
Erythrocytes	:	60% of total body Fe is present as hemoglobin. Each molecule of hemoglobin contains 4 atoms of Fe. 104 mg/100 ml
Plasma	:	Present as transferrin

Tissues

Liver contains 26% of total body Fe

Content in other tissues/body fluids: 14%.

- Present in liver as ferritin (physiological) and hemosiderin (pathological) and in muscles as myoglobin.

ROLE/ESSENTIALITY [50,110,118]

- Vital for life.
- Chief function is in the form of hemoglobin for oxygen transport and tissue respiration.
- Role in various enzyme systems involved in electron transport.
- Constituent of cytochromes *a,b,c,f,* P_{450}, cytochrome reductase, catalase and peroxidases.
- Myoglobin in muscles stores necessary oxygen for muscular activity.

DEFICIENCY [118,195]

- **Blocking of:** (*a*) Oxidative reactions, (*b*) Cell respiration, and (*c*) Energy metabolism.
- **Multiple lipid peroxidation:** Hemolysis.
- **Anaemia:** Iron deficiency causes hypochromic, microcytic anaemia. Infants, school-going children and women in reproductive years are more prone to Fe deficiency. Other causes are blood loss due to injury, hemorrhage or parasites and malabsorption syndromes. It may also occur concurrently with Zn deficiency. The symptoms are pallor of mucus membranes, kolionchiya and general weakness.
- **Other symptoms:** Iron deficiency may also exist without anaemia. It impairs muscle function and limits work capacity and is manifested by weakness, fatigue, headache, irritability, angular stomatitis, atrophic lingual papillae, palpitation, sideropenia dysphagia, hypoproteinemia, hypocupremia, hypogonadism, reduced resistance to infections, dwarfism and concurrent deficiency of folic acid. Prenatal Fe deficiency was recently reported to result in increased post-natal blood pressure even though the offsprings had normal dietary Fe levels from birth.[62]

METABOLISM [15,50,200,209]

Absorption

- **Mucosal Block:** Absorption involves translocation from luminal (mucosal) site to contra-luminal (serosal) site in the intestinal epithelium. Absorption from mucosa is relatively rapid vs. transfer from mucosal cells to circulation which is slow. The latter is a rate limiting step (mucosal block).
- **Site:** Absorption takes place mostly from duodenal and proximal jejunal cells.
- **Regulation:** Absorption takes place by an active energy-mediated process which adapts to demand for Fe. It is under genetic control and dependent on protein synthesis.

- **Extent:** Absorption in human brings is approximately 3-5 mg/day. It is more in women vs. men.
- **Diet:** Available dietary Fe, even in deficiency sates, is about 3 mg/day (average intake: 8-18 mg/day). Only about 7 mg Fe/1000 k cal is actually utilized. There are two types of absorbable Fe in diet : (*a*) Heme iron (sources: meat, poultry, fish). Absorption from average western diet is estimated to be 1-3 mg/day. It is independent of other dietary constituents. (*b*) Non-heme iron (sources: vegetables, wheat, corn). While ascorbate and S containing aminoacids promote absorption, presence of tannates, phosphates, calcium, bran, fibre, chelates (*e.g.*, EDTA used in food preservatives) hinder absorption. Absorption of non-heme Fe is sensitive to the blocking substances in diet.
- **Antagonistic interactions:** Many studies report that high intakes of iron can interfere with the utilization of other trace elements (*e.g.*, Zn, Cu, Cr) and its low intake promotes absorption of some toxic elements (*e.g.*, Cd, Pb). The results of such studies, however, are in disagreement with one another to (*a*) the magnitude of Fe effect and (*b*) its practical relevance for human nutrition.

Storage/Binding/Metabolism

- Most of the absorbed Fe (both heme and non-heme) goes to common pool. Intracellular Fe is temporarily stored as ferritin to be released in next few hours. Iron-binding capacity of ferritin is frequently exceeded. Ferritin is degraded to hemosidrin which accumulates in lysosomes.
- It enters the portal system (unbound or following non-specific binding to albumin). More than 99% of Fe in plasma is bound to transferrin. It is rapidly removed by hepatocytes.
- Internal distribution depends on interaction between proteins and transferrin receptors. Absence of transferrin is a genetic defect. This may be manifested by (*a*) over loading of some tissues (*e.g.*, liver) with Fe and (*b*) inadequate delivery to RBCs resulting in Fe deficiency anaemia.
- Biological half life : 10-20 years.
- ***Useful indices for Fe status:*** (*a*) Ratio of serum transferrin : transaminase activity. (*b*) Serum Fe concentration, and (*c*) Total iron-binding capacity (TIBC).

Excretion

- ***Conservation:*** A unique feature for this vital element is its limited loss : only 10% per year or approx. 1 mg/day. It is need based : in Fe-deficiency anaemia, it is reduced to 0.5 mg/day and in Fe overload increased to 5 mg/day.
- ***Routes:*** Through feces, urine and milk. There is some dermal and menstrual loss.

INTAKE/REQUIREMENTS [118,209]

Intake	**Fe mg/day**
Mean (Range) intake	13 (8-18)

Recommended Dietary Allowance (RDA)		
Infants upto	6 months	10
	6 months to 1 year	15
Children	1-10 years	10-15
	11-18 years	18
Adults	19-50 years Males	10
	Females	18

Additional supplementation of Fe 30-60 mg/day is required for pregnant and lactating women. Loss during lactation is 1 mg/day. This amount can not be met by diet.

GUIDELINE VALUES [118,209]

Occupational Exposure Limit

(40-hour work week)

Elemental Fe:	6 mg/m³
Organic Fe:	8 mg/m³

Drinking water

Maximum permissible limit (India, USA)	0.3 mg/L
Toxic human intake	> 200 mg/day

MEDICINAL USES [118,195]

- Supplementation in Fe deficiency states (anaemia) and when there is more demand (pregnancy, hemorrhage).
- Iron supplements should be given by oral route. Parenteral use should be avoided as far as possible.
- Mere supplementation is not enough. Other factors *e.g.*, cause of deficiency, total iron binding capacity (TIBC), proper utilization etc. should also be looked into.
- Self-medication and indiscriminate use of Fe-containing tonics may be harmful. Iron binding proteins *e.g.*, transferrin are bacteriostatic *in vitro*. This property is lost when these proteins are saturated with Fe predisposing the user to infection.

TOXICITY 15,50,79,118,197,209

Sources of Exposure

- Content in Earth's crust : 4.7%
- Common ores : Hematite, FeO_3, Magnetite, Fe_3O_4, Limonite, FeO (OH), Pyrite, FeS_2, and Boronite, Cu_6FeS_4.
- From uses of alloy steel in:
  - Construction work
  - Machines/Tools
  - Transportation
- Medicinal use

Symptoms

Acute toxicity following overdose of medicinal Fe-preparations is manifested by hemorrhagic gastritis, acidosis, intravascular clotting and fatal shock. Iron overload is associated with **hemochromatosis** and **hemosiderosis**. The latter is caused by deposition of hemosiderin (an Fe containing substance released during splitting of hematin following phagocytic digestion of old erythrocyte). The symptoms include pigmentation of skin, liver and pancreas, cirrhosis and **bronze diabetes**. Excessive use of Fe hematinics has been reported to cause (*a*) **sideroblastic anaemias**, (*b*) increased incidence of **infections** and **stomach cancer**, and (*c*) **porphyria cutaena tarda.**

SYSTEMIC EFFECTS

1. ***Liver:*** Hepatic Fe levels are elevated in hemochromatosis (with visible hemosiderin deposits) and reduced alcoholic fatty and non-fatty cirrhosis. Serum Fe levels show rise in infective hepatitis and all types of jaundice (obstructive, non-obstructive and hemolytic). Iron is a major constituent of biliary calculi.
2. ***Kidney:*** Significantly lower plasma Fe concentrations are observed in nephrosis patients vs. healthy subjects.
3. ***Nervous system:*** Experimental epilepsy has been induced in rats and cats by ferric chloride injection into the isocortex. **Post-menopausal Parkinsonism** has been linked to Fe overload in brain tissue. Patients of endogenous psychosis showed elevated Fe concentrations in caudate nucleus. Neurological manifestations of Fe deficiency include headache, fatigue, irritability, restless legs **(Ekboms' syndrome)** etc. Mental retardation is associated with low-Fe status (hemoglobin, plasma ferritin, TIBC).
4. ***Cardiovascular system:*** While deficiency causes **anaemia,** excess results in platelet aggregation, **hemochromatosis**, catalysis free-radical generation (OH) and cell damage. Marked alterations occur in serum Fe during first 7 days of myocardial infarction.

5. ***Respiratory system:*** Excess Fe enhances production of ${}^{\cdot}OH$ and $O_2^{\cdot -}$ radicals and causes peroxidative damage to endothelial cells of lungs.
6. ***Infectious diseases:*** Though serum Fe levels decrease in infectious diseases, the values are elevated in infective hepatitis with a concurrent rise in total iron-binding capacity (TIBC). **Porphyria cutanea tarda** is linked to Fe overload. It is characterized by photosensitivity, blistering, scattered pigmentation of skin. Depleted serum Fe and anaemia are observed in cases of leprosy and elevated serum Fe values in leucoderma patients.
7. ***Reproductive system:*** Low serum Fe levels are observed from second trimester of pregnancy because of its transfer across placenta to the fetus. Iron supplements are needed to reduce its deficiency in pregnant women and overcome symptoms of anaemia and premature births. While estrogenic activity is inhibited and myotrophic activity of testosterone is depressed by Fe, no appreciable effects were noted on androgenic activity. There is some experimental evidence to indicate that Fe salts may cause irreversible damage to testes and accessary sexual organs resulting in sterility in rats.
8. ***Immune function:*** Both deficiency and overload of this element exert adverse effect on immune function. While severe Fe deficiency inhibits cell-mediated immune responses, no discernible effects were seen on phagocytosis and humoral activity. Iron overload impairs phagocytosis with 40-50% increase in infection episodes. Parenteral administration of Fe promotes bacterial multiplication, aggravates infection which may be lethal.
9. ***Carcinogenic effects:*** Iron promotes cancer-inducing action of carcinogenic agents (Fe particles serve as carriers) and Fe itself is a suspected carcinogen. Fats, heated to 300 °C in contact with iron fillings or in an iron vessel, acquire this property. When a carcinogen is painted on skin, it results in epidermal loss of Fe within 10 days (upto 50%) which is aggravated by continued application. Hepatic tumours are associated with marked reduction in Fe-containing enzymes: catalase and cytochrome P_{450}. Excess following self medication or occupational exposure leads to higher incidence of cancers of the stomach and lungs. The risk is further aggravated in smokers.

MECHANISM OF TOXICITY [15,50,118]

It causes cytotoxic effects by

- Enhanced production of hydroxyl radicals (most potent oxidizing agents existing in aqueous medium).
- Peroxidation of lysosomal membranes.
- Depolymerisation of hyaluronate.
- Platelet aggregation and release of serotonin.

TREATMENT [15,118]

- **Chelation therapy:** Desferrioxamine (DFO) is the specific chelating agent for Fe poisoning. The doses are 15 mg/kg/h by intravenous route or 40-90 mg/kg by deep intramuscular injection. The complex formed between Fe and DFO is very stable. This ensures reduction of extracellular free Fe concentrations and less damage to enzyme systems and cell membranes.

- **Supportive measures:** These include exchange transfusions, hemodialysis, gastrotomy and constant monitoring for hypovolemia, prothrombin time, transaminase and creatinine levels.

KRYPTON (Kr)

CATEGORY

Inert gas. Not reported in human body.

LATHANUM (La)

CATEGORY

Non-essential accumulative trace element.

DISTRIBUTION IN ECOSYSTEM [118]

	La ppm
Earth's crust	30.0
Soil	27.4

HUMAN BODY [36,93,193]

Presence has been reported in blood, bones, brain, heart, kidneys, liver, lungs, lymph nodes, muscles, ovary, placenta, tooth enamel, urine, skin, hair and nails.

ROLE/ESSENTIALITY

Lanthanum is not an essential element. It has no nutritional or physiological role in the human body and there is no known deficiency syndrome for this element.

METABOLISM [118]

Absorption of La from gastro-intestinal tract is very poor. Significant absorption may occur following inhalatory or dermal exposure in occupational setting. The element has a preferential intra-cellular distribution. Following absorption, La competes for or displaces Ca^{2+} from its binding site and acts as a biological antagonist. It gets bound to sarcoplasmic reticulum of muscle cells and to mitochondrial membrane cells in hepatocytes. It mimics actions of Ca^{2+} by activating calmodulin or camodulin-like proteins, interacts with actin, prevents tubule formation and causes alterations in enzyme activities. Its biological half-life is quite long.

MEDICINAL USES [118]

- Lanthanum and other lanthanides are suggested to have therapeutic utility in the management of arthritis because of its following properties : Inhibition of (*a*) Lymphocyte activation, (*b*) Stimulation-mediated cell secretion, (*c*) Neutrophil chemotaxis and aggrevation, and (*d*) Collagenase. Stabilization of collagen fibrils.
- Experimental evidence indicates anti-tumour activity in La : (*a*) Ascites and HeLa cells *in vitro*, (*b*) Sarcomas in rats, (*c*) Lymphatic leukemia and lymphosarcomas in mice. Reports for utility in human beings are not available. Alterations in cell membrane permeability, disruption of membrane potential and tumour metabolism of Ca^{2+} and Mg^{2+} ions are the mechanisms suggested for its anti-tumour activity.

TOXICITY [118]

It has low toxicity. Skin/lung granulomas and pneumoconiosis have been observed after chronic occupational exposure. These include effects on respiratory system, muscles (smooth and cardiac) and axonal activity.

LEAD (Pb)

CATEGORY

- Non-essential accumulative ultra-trace element.

DISTRIBUTION IN ECOSYSTEM [111,125,208,209]

AIR

		Pb ng/m^3
Remote areas (Greenland)	:	15-22
North America	:	2700
Europe	:	120
North India	:	25-1677
Air borne particulate matter of urban Coimbatore (India) was found to be very high in an industrial area	:	Mean 481, Highest 2147

Intakes between 1.5 and 30 μg/day by inhalation have been reported from rural and urban areas in UK.

WATER

Domestic water (Mean Pb content: 10-20 μg/L) may make a significant contribution to the intake of Pb. The metal may get mobilized into ground water from the soil under acidic conditions. Consumption and use of such water should be restricted to protect public health.

SOIL

Surface soil	**Pb mg/kg**
Mean	30
Range	9-84

Uptake of Pb and its entry in food chain is increased by acidic conditions of soil. Agricultural practices, waste disposal and varied human activities also exert influence.

PLANT FOODS [118]

		Pb mg/kgf (fresh weight)
Low 35-200 μg/kg	Cereals	0.035-0.42
	Potatoes	0.09
	Vegetable and fruits	0.07-0.2
High 300-730 μg/kg	Mushrooms	0.3
	Tea	0.73

Acidic foods, tomato juice, fruit juice, cola drinks, pickles, cider, illicit liquor may contain high concentrations of lead possibly from dusty environment, cans and containers.

ANIMAL FOODS [118]

Milk and milk products	9-20 μg/L
Fish	10-30 μg/kg (fresh weight)
Esters and organ meats (Liver, Kidney)	1 mg/kg f

Some fishes may have very high Pcb concentration of lead (upto 500 μg/kgf).

MICROORGANISMS [118]

Biomethylating organisms

Pseudomonas

Acinobacter

Flavobacterium

Aeromonas

HUMAN BODY [50,93,158]

Whole Body Content

- 1.7 ppm
- Content in average adult man (60 kg) : approx. 120-130 mg

DISTRIBUTION

- Distributed in at least 45 human tissues and body fluids including blood, all vital organs (brain, heart, liver, kidneys, lungs), bones, skin etc. About 90% of the total body burden of Pb is found in skeleton.

	Pb µg/L
■ **Blood**	
Erythrocytes	150-610 (mean : 460)
Plasma	120-180 (mean : 130)
	µg/g ash
■ **Skin**	17-46
■ **Vital organs**	
Brain	0.075-0.40
Liver	94-150 (mean : 132)
Lungs	28-82 (mean : 55)
Kidneys	36-140

ROLE/ESSENTIALITY [59,209]

- No known function *per se* or requirement for the function of any enzyme or essential metabolite pathway.
- No known level of exposure below which Pb is harmless.
- Some evidence of essentiality has, however, been shown in rats fed Pb-depleted diets (10-30 μg/kg) for several generations. The symptoms include growth depression, microcytic anaemia with reduction in hemoglobin (23%) and MCV (28%). Depletion in pregnant mothers induced growth retardation (11-20%), reduced blood Fe levels (increased TIBC) and caused hematological changes.

DEFICIENCY

No human deficiency syndrome reported.

METABOLISM [15,50,118,209]

Absorption

(*a*) **Oral**

– Absorption of ingested Pb from gastrointestinal tract is poor (5-15%)

– It is influenced by several factors:

Age: Higher absorption in young children (upto 40%) vs. adults (10%).

Chemical form and solubility: Compounds which are more soluble (*e.g.*, chloride, oxide, acetate) are better absorbed vs. those which are less soluble (*e.g.*, carbonates, chromates, mephides, sulphates).

Diet: Absorption is facilitated by fasting, presence of ascorbic acid, SH-containing amino acids, bile acids and some nutritional deficiencies (Ca, Fe, Vitamin D) and inhibited by ethanol, high phytate, fat, Ca, PO_4, Fe and Mg content in diet which compete for the same carrier sites as Pb. Increased absorption occurs in deficiency states (Ca, Fe, Vitamin D). Larger amounts of Pb are absorbed from liquid diets; experimental animals given liquid diets (*e.g.*, milk) as their only source of food have been shown to result in enhanced absorption and retention of Pb.

(*b*) **Inhalation**

Pulmonary absorption is an important route in view of high concentrations of Pb in ambient air due to vehicular pollution (vapours and particulate matter/dust suspended in atmosphere). It is a two-part process (*i*) deposition in deeper parts of the respiratory tract and (*ii*) absorption of the deposited fraction. The magnitude and rate of absorption is influenced by concentrations in ambient air, respiratory volume and distribution in the respiratory tract. Particle size is a significant determinant; larger particles are cleared in the upper respiratory tract by ciliated epithelial cells, finer particles reach lower respiratory tract where a substantial part (90%) is absorbed or cleared by macrophages and some part retained in alveoli of lungs.

(*c*) **Skin**

Cutaneous absorption for Pb is insignificant but fair amount of lipid-soluble compounds (*e.g.*, tetra ethyl lead) may get absorbed through intact skin.

Distribution/Metabolism

Nearly all of the circulating inorganic Pb (99%) is in erythrocytes (mainly bound to δ-amino levulinic dehydratase) and plasma levels rise only when blood concentrations are very high. Binding occurs mainly with proteins containing free SH groups (*e.g.*, metalothionein which contains cysteine) and relatively less stable complexes are formed with other side chains of amino acids (*e.g.*, lysine, tyrosine). Among the tissues, maximum retention occurs in bones and teeth (> 90%) followed by moderate amounts in liver and kidneys. It is found in nuclei, mitochondria and cell membranes. It crosses both blood-brain and placental barriers. High concentrations are reported in the cortical grey matter and basal ganglia in the brain. Maternal and cord blood values show a direct correlation and there is substantial fetal uptake by 22 weeks of gestation. Tracer studies revealed the following pattern for Pb retention:

(*i*) *Blood:* very short half-life (hour/days). Higher values (1-2 months) have also been reported.

(*ii*) *Soft tissues:* medium half-life (weeks)

(*iii*) *Skeleton:* very long half-life (months/years). Half-life in bones has been reported upto 20-30 years.

Excretion

A substantial part of the ingested Pb (80-90%) is excreted in feces which includes unabsorbed metal plus some amount excreted in bile. Excretion also occurs through urine, sweat, milk, hair and nails. Renal excretion is not substantial but it is important as urinary Pb concentrations parallel plasma levels and so provide a good bioindicator for monitoring Pb status and toxicity.

INTAKE/REQUIREMENTS [15,118,209]

	µg per day
■ Dietary intake (approx. 35% from bread, cereals and beverages)	20-300
■ Higher intake values reported from India	>500
■ Intake from drinking water	20-30
■ Intake by inhalatory route	1.5-30

- Tolerable weekly intake — 20 μg/kg body weight (Max. 3 mg per person)
- No known minimum requirement levels as evidence for its nutritional essentiality is not sufficient.

GUIDELINE VALUES [118,209]

- National air quality standard (India) — 0.75 μg/m^3
- Drinking water
  - Permissible limit (WHO) — 0.05 mg/l
  - National water quality standard (India) — 0.05 mg/l
- Occupational exposure limit (OEL) in air for 40-h work week — 0.10 - 0.15 mg/m^3
- Blood — 150 - 300 μg/l
- Urine Pb — 150 μg/g creatinine
- Urine ALA — 15 μg/l (for women < 45 yr. 6 μg/l)
- Hair Pb — 20 μg/l
- CEC guideline for Pb in gasoline — 0.15-0.40 g/l
- Paints (Germany) Pb — 1%
- Listed by EP under hazardous waste category

MEDICINAL/COSMETIC USES [5,122,123,168,209]

- Lead carbonate is depilatory.
- Lead acetate is incorporated in hair dyes
- Some traditional calcined preparations of this toxic metal are used for therapeutic effects in Indian systems of medicine. Investigations on Ayurvedic *Nag Bhasma* and Unani *Kushta Surb* revealed that these drugs were tolerated at much higher doses vs. the known toxic effects of Pb and its compounds. Besides anticataleptic, anti-aggressive and glycogen sparing (anti-fatigue) actions were observed following administration of these preparations in rats and mice. Some toxic effects were, however, noted in animals on 6-months treatment schedule at high doses. Another Unani preparation *Kushta-e-Musallus* also exhibited interesting neuro-behavioural properties with adequate margin of safety.

TOXICITY [15,42,50,107,117,118,200,209]

Sources of Exposure/Contamination

From extensive uses in:

(*a*) petrol/gasoline: tetraethyl lead as anti-knock agent. Use of deleaded petrol has considerably reduced such exposure.

(*b*) paints: dried chips from walls may contain 5-40% Pb. US standard for paints used on toys, furniture, dwellings: < 1% Pb.

(*c*) storage batteries

(*d*) ammunition

(*e*) glassware/ceramics

(*f*) printing press

(*g*) ball-bearing alloys

(*h*) rubber industry

(*i*) radiation protection

Metal contamination of soils and crops from a Pb/Zn mine spill has recently been reported from South China. Consumption of such crop may be hazardous to health.[107]

Toxicity depends on magnitude, route and duration of exposure as while the metal affects all systems, the effects are more pronounced on three systems:

(*i*) Haemopoietic system

(*ii*) Nervous system

(*iii*) Renal system

SYSTEMIC EFFECTS [3,15,41,80,118,200,209]

1. ***Liver:*** Increased Pb content was reported in hemochromatosis (upto 7 times the control value), Laennec's cirrhosis and Wilson's disease. Experimental Pb toxicity has been shown to decrease hepatic ascorbic acid content in rats fed on-low or high-protein diet.

2. ***Gastro-intestinal system:*** Symptoms of Pb toxicity include severe colic (umbilical region), vomiting (milky white in case of Pb chloride poisoning), distressing intestinal spasm, constipation or diarrhoea (black stools in case of Pb sulphide poisoning), anorexia, metallic taste and blue lines on gums.

3. ***Cardiovascular system:*** High blood Pb concentration (> 30 μg/dl) may lead to ECG changes and hypertension. The association of hypertensive effect of Pb is stronger for elderly males (40-50 years) vs. younger people and females and more for systolic vs. diastolic BP. The biochemical and physiological mechanisms involved in hypertensive effects of Pb have not been fully elucidated. Possibilities include: (*a*) vascular reactivity, (*b*) sympathetic tone, (*c*) renin-angiotensin system, and (*d*) intra-cellular Ca^{2+} levels.

4. ***Hemopoietic system:*** Lead interacts with several essential elements (particularly Ca and Fe) and affects all steps in haeme synthesis with primary effect on immature erythrocytes. It causes : (*a*) reduction in uptake and utilization of Fe, (*b*) increase in biodegradation of haeme, (*c*) hemolysis of erythrocytes, (*d*) decrease in concentration of circulating hemoglobin, (*e*) reduction in mean life span of circulating RBCs in both children and adults, (*f*) anaemia with reticulocytosis, (*g*) basophilic stippling of erythroblastic cells due to aggregation of RNA (blood Pb : > 80 μg/dl), and (*h*) accumulation of δ-aminolevulinic acid dehydratase (δ-ALAD) and Zn protoporphyrin (ZPP) in RBCs.

5. ***Kidney:*** Renal Pb content increases with intake. Acute or chronic nephropathy results depending on dose and duration of exposure. Acute exposure causes reversible tubular damage and impaired reabsorption. This is manifested by glycosuria, aminoaciduria, hyperphosphaturia, hypophosphataemia, acidosis and presence of nuclear inclusion bodies in urinary sediments. Prolonged exposure may lead to irreversible interstitial fibrosis, contracted kidneys, tubular-vascular lesions, nephrosclerosis, glomerular atrophy, hyaline degeneration of vessels and renal failure.

6. ***Nervous system:*** Among all organs, brain is most sensitive to Pb exposure resulting in electrophysiological (EEG), neurochemical (neuro transmitter function, acetylcholine, noradrenaline, dopamine, serotonin, GABA, Ca), and neuro behavioural (neuromuscular and cognitive) effects. Infants/children are more sensitive to Pb toxicity vs. adults; 65% mortality reported in untreated cases with cerebral encephalopathy. This is due to: (*a*) greater absorption of ingested Pb, (*b*) immature blood-brain barrier and (*c*) a nervous system which is still under development. Exposure in adults (occupational or accidental) is largely manifested by peripheral neuropathy. **Peripheral neuropathy** primarily affects the large myelinated nerve fibres with **demyelination** and **axonal degeneration**. The effects may be subtle or serious in nature. The former include: headache, insomnia, nervousness, psychosis, mood fluctuations, lack of concentration, **learning disability, low I.Q.**, slowing of nerve conduction velocity, lassitude, fatigue etc. The clinical profile may shift to serious effects: encephalopathy with predominant motor features **(wrist and foot drop)**, cerebral oedema, ataxia, paralysis of extensor/flexor muscles, tremours, aggressive episodes and mania. Degenerative changes are observed in motor neurons and their axons.

approximately 25% mortality occurs in cases with **cerebral oedema** due to increased cranial pressure. Fetal exposure to Pb has been reported to affect neuro-behavioural parameters in children, EEG profile and hearing threshold. Developing nervous system is the most sensitive target organ system.

Children recovering from Pb **encephalopathy** may show symptoms of **mental retardation**, epilepsy and in some cases **cortical blindness**. Precise threshold blood Pb levels have not been established but some indicators are available. No evidence of cognitive dysfunction is discernible at levels < 25 μg/dl Pb. Low IQ values are observed when Pb concentrations exceed this limit. Levels > 30-50 μg/dl are associated with **cognitive dysfunction** and so necessitate remedial measures.

7. ***Reproductive system:*** Exposure to Pb is reported to shorten gestation period, cause spontaneous abortions, and reduce fetal growth and size. Both male and female reproductive system are adversely affected. This is evidenced by negative effects on sperm count, hormone chemistry and fetal growth and development (including mental development). A study on 18 infertile and 38 men of known fertility, however, revealed no significant differences in their blood Pb levels.

8. ***Immune Function:*** Lead produces adverse effects on immune function. These effects are observed at very low exposure levels at which other systemic effects are not discernible. Studies in mice and rats revealed following alterations:

Decrease	*Increase*
(*a*) Weight of thymus gland	(*a*) Concanvalin A activity
(*b*) Serum immunoglobulin levels	(*b*) Passive cutaneous anaphylaxis to ovalbumin
(*c*) T cell-dependent antibody response	(*c*) Susceptibility to endotoxins and infectious agents
(*d*) B-cell rosetting	
(*e*) Delayed hypersensitivity to sheep RBCs	
(*f*) Phagocytic activity	

While cell-mediated immunity and reticuloendothelial functions are moderately affected, the action of Pb on humoral response is more pronounced. A significant negative correlation has been reported between blood Pb concentrations and serum levels of complement C_3 and IgG on exposed workers. The effects depend on the type of Pb salt, dose and duration of exposure.

9. ***Carcinogenicity:*** Lead is reported to be mutagenic and genotoxic. It causes disturbance in enzymatic functions inducing chromosomal aberrations. There is considerable experimental evidence to show its carcinogenic effects. Lead compounds *e.g.*, acetate, subacetate and phosphate, when injected or administered in diet, were shown to induce renal tumours in rodents. The carcinogenic effects were observed at very high doses of Pb in animals with obvious symptoms of Pb toxicity with appearance of nuclear inclusion bodies in renal cells. Higher human incidence of cancer mortality (gastrointestinal tract, respiratory and renal cancers) has been reported following long-term occupational exposure among Pb smelter and battery plant workers. The IARC and US-EPA have advised for a cautious approach and further investigations on this aspect.

10. ***Teratogenicity:*** The metal crosses placental barrier and reaches fetus following intragastric or chronic inhalatory exposure. The effects observed in mice, rats, rabbits and hamsters include increased embryonic mortality, reduced fetal size, impaired post-natal development and teratogenicity. Human studies revealed reduced gestation period and frequent abortions. While minor fetal malformations are suspected in exposed women, but the evidence for human teratogenicity is not conclusive. Mental development index (MDI), however, link maternal Pb levels as low as 10-15 μg/dl with growth retardation, deficient neurobehavioural performance and impaired post-natal development in children.

MECHANISMS OF TOXICITY [15,99,118]

(*a*) Interference with enzymes involved in haeme synthesis *e.g.*, δ-aminolevulinic acid synthetase (ALAS), δ-aminolevulinic acid dehydratase (ALAD), ferrochelatase etc. and reduction in haemoprotein biosynthesis. In a recent study from Korea, an overall prevalence of ALAD 1-2/2-2 genotype was found to be 9.2% and its association was shown with low Zn protoporphysin (ZPP) and high blood Pb levels.[100]

(*b*) Oxidative damage to erythrocyte membrane.

(*c*) Depression of serum dihydrocholecalciferol, possibly through the inhibition of cytochrome P_{450}.

(*d*) Involvement of Ca, cholinergic, monaminergic (dopamine, norepinephrine, 5 hydroxytryptamine) and GABAergic system has been suggested in the neurotoxic effects of Pb.

(*e*) Altered permeability of brain capillaries, segmental demylination and axonal degeneration of peripheral motor nerves.

(*f*) Hypertensive and renal effects are mediated through renin angiotensin system.

DIAGNOSTIC FEATURES [15,79,118,209]

Diagnosis of Pb poisoning is based on :

1. ***History:*** Pb exposure, dose, route etc.
2. ***Clinical presentation:*** Among the signs and symptoms, described under systemic effects, the following are diagnostic:
   - Ashen face, pallor on lips, black Pb lines on gums.
   - Colic in umbilical region, milky vomitus, black stools
   - Renal dysfunction
   - Hypertension, anaemia
   - Poor muscle tone, stooping posture, wrist and foot drop, low IQ in children: decrement by 2-5 points (blood Pb: 20-70 μg/dl).
3. ***Laboratory investigations:***

– **Gastrointestinal tract/ Bones:** Detection of unabsorbed Pb in GIT by X-ray and measurement of Pb in long bones by X-ray fluorescence technique.

– **Blood examination:**

Pb level > 25 μg/dl

Inhibition of δ ALAD activity

Accumulation of ZPP in erythrocytes

Basophilic stippling of erythrocytes

(blood Pb : > 80 μg/dl)

Lead concentrations in umbilical cord blood and dentine of shed teeth have been used as indices for childhood Pb exposure.

– ***Urine examination:***

Normal: < 80 μg Pb/l (Safe levels : 52 μg/l)

Poisoning cases: 150-300 μg Pb/l

(Toxic : 107 μg/l, Dangerous: 175 μg/l and above)

Detection of inclusion bodies in urinary sediments.

– ***Organs/Tissues:*** Inclusion bodies in cord cells, proximal tubular cells of kidneys, osteoblasts, brain glial cells. This is a protective mechanism to maintain concentrations in cytoplasm at low level.

- ***$CaNa_2$, EDTA mobilisation test :*** It is a good indicator for body burden of Pb. A single dose of Ca Na_2 EDTA (50 μg/kg i.v.) is given and urinary samples collected hourly for 8 hours.

$$\text{If the ratio : } \frac{\text{Pb excreted (μg)}}{\text{Chelating agent (mg)}} \text{ is} > 0.6$$

in children, the test is positive indicating Pb toxicity. This test is not suitable for symptomatic patients and those with blood Pb values > 100 μg/l. Experimental studies in rats on chronic low level Pb exposure revealed that Ca Na_2 EDTA may double brain Pb concentrations and so safety of the test is doubtful. Such patients require proper treatment.

- ***Post-mortem examination:*** Black lines on diaphysis of epiphyseal cartilage of long bones (blood Pb: > 60 μg/dl). Neurological lesions.

TREATMENT [15,99,118]

(*a*) Chelation Therapy:

Indications:

- Acute encephalopathy
- Classic symptomatic cases (plumbism)
- Asymptomatic cases with high blood Pb levels (> 50-60 μg/dl)

Agents:

- Disodium calcium EDTA, combination of dimercaprol with $CaNa_2$ EDTA, D-penicillinamine, unithiol, meso 2,3 dimercaptosuccinic acid (DMSA, Succimer), and sodium salt of 2,3 dimercapto 1 propane sulfonate (DMPS, Dimval) have been used for the treatment of Pb poisoning.

Ca Na_2 EDTA, given orally, may enhance absorption of Pb. It is given at 75 mg/kg by i.m. injection (or sometimes slow i.v. injection) in 2 divided doses for 5 days. The total dose during the course of treatment should not exceed 500 mg/kg. D penicillinamine administered p.o. can mobilize Pb from bones. Combined therapy with Ca Na_2 EDTA and BAL is quite effective in preventing rapid mobilization of Pb into blood. Agents of first and second choice are DMSA and DMPS, respectively

(*b*) Symptomatic therapy and supportive measures:

- Monitoring of blood Pb levels for determination of renal flow. Generous flow of urine must be maintained.
- Symptomatic treatment for seizures, cerebral edema and encephalopathy: Diazepam, mannitol, dexamethasone etc. may be used. Calcium gluconate is reported to be more effective in colic vs. morphine. Procaine or lidocaine may be added during i.m. injection of chelating agents to reduce pain.

– Diet with high Ca, low PO_4 and adequate Fe content

– Dust control measures.

LITHIUM (Li)

CATEGORY

Possibly essential trace element.

DISTRIBUTION IN ECOSYSTEM [118,209]

AIR

Not available

WATER

Sea water	180 ppb
Drinking water	5-80 μg/L

SOIL	**Li mg/kg**
Content in soil shows	
wide variations	< 10 to > 100
Average concentration	30

PLANTS	**Li μg/g**
Wide species/soil variations	0.4 to > 1000
Leguminous plants	50

HUMAN BODY [93,158,209]

Whole Body Content

- 0.04 ppm
- Content in average adult man (60 kg) : 2.2 mg

Distribution

Presence of Li has been reported in at least 18 human tissues and body fluids including blood and all vital organs. Concentrations in human and animal tissues range between 2 and 200 n/kg wet weight. Reported reference concentrations in human tissues/body fluids are as follows: Whole blood 0.4 - 1 μg/l, Serum 0.2 - 0.8 μg/l, milk < 1 μg/l, urine 25-100 μg/day, hair 10-100 μg/kg.

ROLE/ESSENTIALITY [118,178,200,209]

- Li belongs to the same group (Ia) of elements as the indispensable Na and K.
- Li ions mimic the action of Na in many ways and can replace Na in nerve, muscle and erythrocyte preparations to some extent.

- Role in neurotransmission.
- Role in immune function: Li enhances DNA-synthesis, lymphocyte proliferation, thymidine uptake, interleukin II and helper cell activity and reverses activity of suppressor cells obtained from patients with immune deficiency or plaque-forming cell activity in culture.
- Insulin-mimetic properties
- **Biochemical Effects:**

  (*i*) Li cation is very stable. Though it does not directly participate in redox reactions, it reacts with cyclic polyethers, polypeptides and proteins.

  (*ii*) Influences inositol phosphate reactions.

  (*iii*) It affects glycolytic pathways and citric acid cycle.

  (*iv*) At the beginning of Li therapy the following show increased levels in brain :

  (*a*) glucose 6 phosphate,

  (*b*) α-ketoglucotarate

  (*c*) 6-phosphogluconate

  (*d*) glutamate

  (*e*) glycogen

  Serum Mg concentrations are also elevated. Later all these alterations are normalized.

  (*v*) GABA transaminase activity is inhibited following Li treatment resulting in accumulation of GABA in brain.

  (*vi*) Li increases brain norepinephrine levels and enhances its deamination.

  (*vii*) It facilitates binding of serotonin to receptors in brain and increases release of 5-HT from hippocampus but not from cortex.

DEFICIENCY [93,113,118,200,209]

Deficiency syndromes have been demonstrated in rats and goats on very low Li intake levels with following symptoms:

(*a*) higher abortion rates and post-partum mortality.

(*b*) reduced birth weight and weight gain during first 6 months.

Epidemiological studies in human populations in USA revealed that low Li content in drinking water resulted in:

(*a*) higher mortality rate from heart disease.

(*b*) more hospital admissions for mental ailments.

METABOLISM

Detailed reports are not available. Chief route of excretion is through urine.

MEDICINAL USES [79,80,192,200,209]

(*a*) Lithium carbonate has been used worldwide in psychiatric medicine for the prophylaxis and treatment of **Maniac Depressive Psychosis (MDP)**. Lithium is neither sedative nor euphoriant, but on prolonged administration, it acts as a mood stabilizer. When given in acute cases, it suppresses maniac episodes in 1-2 weeks. Effective doses (starting dose : 600 mg/day, latter doses, 250-500 mg/day) require close monitoring because of narrow therapeutic index of Li therapy. Chronic toxicity may occur with excessive weight gain and adverse effects on thyroid function. It should not be used in pregnancy. While the precise mechanism of action of Li is not known, the tranquillizing effects are possibly mediated through GABAergic actions. Drug interactions are reported with diazepam, haloperidol, methyldopa and antiepileptic drugs.

(*b*) Li salts were used earlier for the treatment of many human diseases *e.g.*, thyrotoxicosis, Graves' disease, Huntington's chorea, gout, diabetes, epilepsy etc. but their utility in these ailments is doubtful and so these are no longer used in such cases.

INTAKE/REQUIREMENTS [139,209]

Average intake	Li µg/day
USA	60-70
Turkey	102
Finland	35
Japan	61

As its essentiality is not established, no RDA values have been worked out.

GUIDELINE VALUES [118]

	Li mg/m^3
Occupational exposure level in air	0.025

TOXICITY [77,209]

Plasma levels > 2.5 meq/L produce toxic symptoms and concentrations > 4 meq/L may be fatal. Symptoms include gastro-intestinal, behavioural and cardiovascular abnormalities. Nausea/vomiting/ diarrhoea occur within one hour of acute intoxication. Neurological symptoms may take several hours. These include lethargy, muscular weakness, ataxia, myoclonic jerks, convulsions, delirium, hyperthermia, coma etc. Cardiac abnormalities (T wave inversion in ECG, bradycardia, sinus node arrest), polyuria and respiratory failure may also be observed. The mechanisms involved in toxic effects are displacement of electrolytes (Na, K, Mg, Ca) from intracellular and bone sites, inhibition of the release and uptake of noradrenaline at nerve terminals, reduction of cell-mediated synthesis of c-AMP etc. Specific antidotes are not known and so only symptomatic treatment and supportive measures are taken up in cases of Li poisoning.

LUTETIUM (Lu)

CATEGORY

Non-essential accumulative ultra-trace element.

DISTRIBUTION IN ECOSYSTEMS [118]

Earth's crust	0.5 ppm

HUMAN BODY [93,193]

Presence has been reported in blood and tooth enamel.

ROLE AND TOXICITY [118]

Lutetium is a non-essential element with no known nutritional or physiological role or deficiency disease. Like other lanthanides, it competes for and can displace Ca^{2+} ions, interacts with actin and prevents tubule formation. No reports on toxic manifestations, following exposure to Lu, are available.

MAGNESIUM (Mg)

CATEGORY

Essential bulk element.

DISTRIBUTION IN ECOSYSTEMS [118,142]

AIR

Not available

WATER

River water	4.1 mg/kg

Hardness of water is inversely proportional to BP and incidence of cardiovascular diseases.

SOIL

Content in earth's crust	2%
Higher content in rock vs. soils because of Mg loss during weathering.	
Exchangeable cation available to plants	5-30%

PLANT FOODS [118]

	Mg g/kg
Average content in plants	1-8
Content in plant foods	
Nuts	2.00
Cereals	0.80
Legumes	0.24
Vegetables	0.17
Fruits	0.07

ANIMAL FOODS [118]

Average content in fish and mammals	1.00
Content in animal foods	0.35
Meat	0.27
Dairy products	0.18

HUMAN BODY [14,158,210,211]

Whole Body Content

- 1.3 hundred thousand atoms per billion atoms
- 272-420 mg/kg of body weight
- 0.05% of the total weight of protoplasm
- 0.5 g/kg of fat-free tissues

- 270 ppm
- Content in average adult man (60 kg) 16-25g

Distribution

- Magnesium is present in all living cells. Widely distributed in all tissues and body fluids, presence reported in > 50 tissues and body fluids.
- Approximately 60% of the total body content is present in skeleton (1.1 g/kg wet weight). The remaining 40% is almost entirely present inside the cells; only 1% of this part is in the extracellular fluid.
- **Blood**

	Mg mg/L
Whole blood	18-23
Serum	20
Erythrocytes	5.3-12

- **Tissues**

Content in major tissues/organs e.g. brain, heart, liver, kidney, lungs, spleen etc.	5-13 μg/kg
Ratio between intracellular and extracellular content in soft tissues	10 : 1

ROLE/ESSENTIALITY [110,118,187,192,202,207]

- ***Photosynthesis:*** Magnesium is an essential constituent of chlorophyll in plants which is needed to capture solar energy for the synthesis of organic molecules including food. Oxygen, which is vital for life, appeared in Earth's atmosphere during evolution as a bi-product of photosynthesis.
- ***Enzymes:*** It is a constituent or ionic activator of about 300 mammalian enzymes regulating many physiological processes including NaK ATPase: the enzyme necessary for maintenance of intracellular-extracellular ionic homeostasis. All enzyme reactions, catalyzed by ATP, require Mg. Complex of ATP with Mg is needed for electron transport and normal mitochondrial function. It has a vital role in oxidative phosphorylation, tissue respiration, and bioenergetic mechanisms.
- ***Heart:*** The element has gained importance because of its role in cardiovascular function in health and disease by lipid regulation, effect on blood coagulation, thrombus formation, atherosclerosis, ischemic heart disease and stress.

- ***Growth and development:*** As a constituent of bones and teeth, Mg is essential for growth and development.
- ***Physical performance:*** In contrast to Vitamins (A, B_{12} and E), marginal mineral deficiencies impair performance, Magnesium deprivation increases oxygen requirements to complete submaximal exercise and reduces physical performance.
- ***Epilepsy:*** The ratios of serum Mg : Zn levels are reported to be < 1 in healthy subjects and >1 in epileptic patients. Diagnostic significance of these observations has not been elucidated.
- ***Cognitive function:*** Nootropic effects of $MgSO_4$ have been reported in rats and mice.

DEFICIENCY [46,118,187,189,200]

Conditions

Magnesium is abundant in nature and diet. So, under normal circumstances, deficiency is unlikely. Deficiency may, however, occur in following conditions:

(*a*) Alcoholism

(*b*) Kwashiorkor

(*c*) Malabsorption syndrome

(*d*) Diuretics and digitalis therapy

(*e*) Hypercholesterolemia/Atherosclerosis

(*f*) Acute pancreatitis

(*g*) Chronic nephritis

(*h*) Loss of fluids: Hemorrhage, Diarrhoea

(*i*) Idiopathic epilepsy etc.

Deficiency is linked with Ca, P and Vitamin D content in diet. Interrelationship has been reported with Ca and parathyroid hormone.

Symptoms

(*a*) Neuromuscular irritability

(*b*) Convulsions

(*c*) Tetany

(*d*) Behavioural/psychosomatic disturbances

(*e*) Gastric, metabolic and renal disturbances

(*f*) Weakness

(*g*) Cardiovascular ailments: arrhythmias, ischemic heart disease, congestive heart failure, myocardial infarction, mitral valve prolapse, stroke etc.

(*h*) Morphological alterations in thymus gland and lymph nodes resulting in disturbances in immune function.

(*i*) Pre-eclampsia

(*j*) Low levels observed in cervical cancer.

(*k*) Sudden death.

METABOLISM [118,187]

Absorption

Gastro-intestinal absorption of Mg ranges between 12 to 40%. Some of it is secreted back into intestines and partly reabsorbed.

Distribution/Metabolism

Absorbed Mg gets distributed to all tissues and body fluids. Bulk (90%) of it is present in bones and muscles. It is the second-most abundant intracellular cation (99%) following K.

Excretion

Major part (60-90%) is excreted in feces and remaining through urine. Kidney plays main role in regulating Mg content in the body.

INTAKE [118,209]

Dietary Intake	Mg µg/day
Range of dietary intake (IAEA)	190-420
Median dietary intake (WHO)	300
Average American intake	240-480

REQUIREMENTS [118]

Recommended Dietary Allowances (RDA)

Infants	**Mg mg/day**
upto 6 months	40
6 months to 1 year	60
Children	
1-3 years	80
4-6 years	120
7-10 years	170
Adult	
Average adult	350-400
Additional during pregnancy/lactation	150

GUIDELINE VALUES [118]

	Mg mg/m^3
Occupational Exposure Level (OEL) for Mg oxide in air	
Germany	6
USA, UK	10

MEDICINAL USES [56,57,79,115,118,195,207]

1. ***Acidity and constipation***

   Magnesium salts are antacid and $MgSO_4$ is used as a purgative.

2. ***Cardiovascular diseases***

   In recent years, Mg has received great attention for its role and great therapeutic potential in many cardiovascular ailments:

   (*a*) Hypertension

   (*b*) Stroke

   (*c*) Congestive heart failure

   (*d*) Endomyocardial fibrosis

   (*e*) Mitral valve prolapse

   (*f*) Arrhythmias

   (*g*) Ischemic heart disease

   (*h*) Acute myocardial infarction etc.

Epidemiological evidence shows an inverse relationship between hardness of water and Mg content of local soil with the incidence of hypertension, IHD, AMI and sudden death. Clinical enhancement of the hypotensive effect of diuretics is observed by Mg therapy. Experimental studies indicate that Mg depletion results in increased infarct size. Similarly, autopsy reports revealed lower myocardial Mg content in victims living in soft water areas. Further Mg content was found to be lower in cases of IHD and sudden death victims vs. myocardial samples from victims of traumatic death.

Clinical studies with Mg preparations revealed very encouraging results: reduction in ventricular arrhythmias and mortality. The doses of $MgSO_4$ i.v. infusion in cases of IHD are 2g over 30 min followed by 5 g over 12 h and for AMI 22 g in 1 *l* distilled water infused over 48 h as follows:

(*a*) 90 ml/h during first 3h

(*b*) 22 ml/h for next 21h and

(*c*) 11 ml/h for next 24 h. Besides Mg sulphate, other salts *e.g.*, oxide, chloride, acetate, gluconate and lactate are also used for therapy.

The mechanisms whereby Mg elicits beneficial effect in cardiovascular diseases include its following properties/actions:

(*a*) Vasodilatory/Hypotensive effects.

(*b*) Reduction in excessive secretion of catecholamines.

(*c*) Antiarrhythmic action (direct effect and also through effect on Ca and K metabolism).

(*d*) Anticoagulant, fibrinolytic and antithrombotic actions.

(*e*) Protection against stress/anxiety.

3. ***Pre eclampsia/toxemia of pregnancy:*** Low Mg levels enhance the vasoconstrictor response to neurohumoral agents *e.g.*, epinephrine, nor-epinephrine, angiotensin II, serotonin, acetylcholine, bradykinin and K. Se, Mg replenishment reduces excitibility of smooth muscles. Parentral Mg alone or in combination with other drugs (ß agonist ritodrine) controls pre-term labour and prolongs pregnancy with no ill effects on neonates except slight hypotonia.
4. ***Other conditions:*** Magnesium has also been reported to be useful in cases of asthma, obstructive lung disease, alcoholism, alcohol withdrawl syndrome, diabetes mellitus, and for euthanesia in veterinary medicine. Good Mg status is associated with reduced diabetes risk and improved insulin status.

TOXICITY [118,187]

Toxicity with Mg seldom occurs following accidental or intentional poisoning, or medicinal overdose. Kidneys handle Mg efficiently under normal conditions keeping serum levels approximately 20 mg/L. Hypermagnesemia may occur in cases of renal impairment/failure. The symptoms include gastrointestinal hyperactivity (nausea, vomiting, diarrhoea), CNS depression (sedation, muscle weakness, reduction in deep tendon reflexes) hypotension and ECG changes. Discontinuation of Mg therapy and symptomatic measures are taken.

MANGANESE (Mn)

CATEGORY

Essential ultra-trace element.

DISTRIBUTION IN ECOSYSTEMS[111,118]

AIR

	Mn ng/m^3
Remote Areas (Greenland)	0.1-16.7
Europe and America	20-850
North India	25-1677

WATER

	Mn µg/L
River water	4.00
Sea water	0.01

A survery of 4 treatment plants and 80 tube-wells at Delhi revealed marginally higher Mn levels vs. the specified Indian standards.[49]

SOIL

	Mn ppm
Mean (Range)	325 (235-458)

PLANT FOODS [118]

	mg/kg f
Cereals	11-34
Vegetable and fruits	0.5-7.4
Tea	15
Mushrooms	734

ANIMAL FOODS [118]

	mg/kg f
Milk/milk products	0.1-1.8 (mean: 0.7)
Meat	0.2-0.3
Organ meats (Liver, Kidney)	10
Fish/Sea food	0.12-4.6

HUMAN BODY [14,93,158]

Whole Body Content

- 170 atoms per billion atoms in the body
- 15.3 million atoms in each cell
- 0.2 ppm
- Content in an average adult man (60 kg) : approx 10-20 mg.

Distribution

- Widely distributed in >50 tissues/body fluids.
- Concentrated in mitochondria and nuclei, nucleotides, DNA and RNA.
- High concentrations in pituitary, gastrointestinal tract tissues, liver, pancreas and kidneys.
- Constituent of hepatic mitochondria
- Constituent of many enzymes.

ROLE [79,118,187,200]

- Essential for formation of connective tissue and bones, skeletal development, growth, reproduction and brain function. It catalyzes the formation of glucosamine-serine linkages during the synthesis of mucopolysaccharides of cartilages.
- **Enzymatic functions:**

(*a*) *As a constituent*

Enzyme	Lack/Deficiency
Arginase	No urea synthesis. Ammonia intoxication
Malic enzyme/pyruvate carboxylase	Citric acid cycle blocked
Superoxide dismutase	Destruction of mitochondria by free-oxygen radicals.

(*b*) *As an activator*

Activator of coenzymes concerned with carbohydrate, protein and fat metabolism.

(*c*) *As a cofactor*

Cofactor of hydrolase, decarboxylase, transferase and several mitochondrial enzymes. Role in synthesis of glycoproteins and proteoglycans.

- Lipotropic action, synthesis of cholesterol and fatty acids. Role in lipogenesis is confirmed by several experimental studies. Mechanisms include its role as a cofactor in steroid biosynthesis, stimulation of enzymes involved in glycolysis and pentose phosphate pathway and through an effect on insulin metabolism. The metabolic site of action appears to be at the stage of formation of farnesyl pyrophosphate from the condensation of geranyl and isopentinyl pyrophosphate. Farensyl pyrophosphatase synthase, the enzyme catalyzing this reaction, is activated by Mn.
- Role suspected but not proved in diabetes mellitus.
- Metabolism of biogenic amines.
- Serum Mn values are elevated in acute coronary occlusion (values show two-fold increase) and viral hepatitis. Estimation of serum Mn levels is reported to be a better criteria for myocardial infarction vs. SGOT determination. Hair Mn slows five-fold increase in Kwashiorkor disease.

DEFICIENCY [78,118,182,187,209]

- Normal diets contain sufficient amounts of Mn, so deficiency is unlikely but deficiency states may occur in children.
- Deficiency syndrome is well documented in animals. Experimental deficiency in mice is reported to cause ultrastructural changes (integrity of cell membranes, swelling of endoplasmic reticulum changes in mitochondria) in renal cells. Deficiency states were not reported in man till 1971 when Hambidge described it in a human volunteer. Concurrent deficiency of Mn and vitamin K in this subject lead to a marked increase in the levels of serum cholesterol, phospholipids and triglycerides. Other symptoms included weight loss, reduced growth of hair and nails, pigment changes, dermatitis, reddening of black hair etc. According to a WHO document, unequivocal evidence for Mn deficiency has not been reported in humans so far.
- Symptoms include:

  (*i*) postural defects, ataxia, motor incoordination, convulsions. Neonatal ataxia may be attributed to improper otolith development. Skeletal abnormalities have been linked to alterations in Mn-dependent enzymes *e.g.*, galacto-transferase and polymerases.

  (*ii*) aplasia or hyperplasia of pancreas.

  (*iii*) abnormal carbohydrate metabolism.

  (*iv*) increased tolerance to intravenous glucose.

  (*v*) hypercholesterolemia

  (*vi*) prothrombin deficiency

  (*vii*) impaired reproductive function, possibly due to defective steroid synthesis, is manifested by menstrual disturbances, azoospermia, reduced fertility, still births.

  (*viii*) dermatitis.

METABOLISM [15,118,209]

Absorption

- ***Oral:*** Though absorption occurs throughout the length of small intestine, only 3-4% of Mn is absorbed through this route. It is not under homeostatic control. So, Mn content in diet or total body burden of this metal apparently have no effect on the rate or extent of absorption. The rate, however, is considerably increased in some physiological and pathological conditions *e.g.*, infancy, pregnancy, iron-deficiency anaemia (upto 7%) and alcoholism.

- ***Inhalation:*** Respiratory tract is an important route for the absorption of Mn.
- ***Skin:*** Organo-manganese compounds may be absorbed through intact skin.

Distribuition/Metabolism

- ***Half-life*** Oral 10 days
  Intravenous 40 days
- ***Binding :*** Most of the absorbed Mn gets bound to α_2 macroglobulin after entry into the portal blood. It is also incorporated in RBCs during erythropoeisis. Some part gets bounds to transferrin following oxidation to Mn^{3+}. It is bound to mitochondria within the cells.
- It is distributed in bound forms to most tissues and body fluids with high concentrations in intestines, liver, pancreas, kidneys and several metalo-enzymes.
- Crosses both the placental and blood-brain barrier to reach fetus and the brain. Half life in brain is longer vs. rest of the body.
- Biogenic amines influence metabolic pathways.

Excretion

- Excretion pattern, which is variable, is believed to maintain homeostasis.
- ***Routes:*** Main route of excretion for inorganic Mn is through bile and feces, marginal excretion occurs through pancreatic juice and kidneys. While urinary excretion for inorganic Mn is only 0.1-1.3% of daily intake, for organomanganese tricarbonyl compounds (used as additives in gasoline) there is substantial renal excretion. A part of the inhaled Mn is cleared by mucociliatory action.
- New-born infants have low capacity to excrete Mn and, therefore, are constitute a high risk group for Mn toxicity.

INTAKE [41,209]

	mg per day
Average intake	3-8
China	7.8
India	8.3
Canada	3.1
New Zealand	2.7
USA	2.9
UK	5.1

Dietary intake depends on the type of diet. A recent WHO publication reported high Mn intake (8.3 mg/day) from Indian diets which are high in foods of plant origin in contrast to very low intake (0.36-1.78 mg/day) from highly-refined hospital diets in USA.

REQUIREMENTS [60,209]

	mg per day
Adults	2.5-5.0

Precise basal requirements are not known and remain to be determined; the range (lower limit to induce deficiency and maximum safe level) indicated for an average adult is, therefore, tentative.

GUIDELINE VALUES [118,209]

	Mn mg/L
■ Drinking water (India)	
Permissible	0.1
Excessive	0.5
■ Occupational exposure limit (OEL) in air for 40-h work week	1-5 mg/m^3
■ Because of small particle size, smoke is more dangerous vs. dust.	
■ Uine Mn	50 μg/l

MEDICINAL USES [12,79,195]

A South African diabetic, who was poorly controlled by insulin, treated himself with alfa-alfa tea extract. The latter is known to be rich in Mn. It was further observed that oral administration of Mn to this patient was effective in restoring normoglycaemia within 3 to 4 hours. This is an isolated report, no other report is available to confirm or refute it.

TOXICITY [15,40,118,200]

Sources of Exposure/Contamination

Elemental Mn is relatively non-toxic. Strong oxidizing compounds *e.g.*, potassium permangnate are very toxic. Though it is considered to be one of the least toxic trace elements (maximum tolerated dose: > 30 mg/day), toxicity may occur from industrial and household usage in:

(*a*) Alloys (including steel)

(*b*) Dry-cell batteries: cases of poisoning have been reported following consumption of well water contaminated from Mn released from discarded batteries.

(*c*) Diesel exhaust filters.

(*d*) Antiknock agents: use of methylcyclopentadienyl Mn tricarbonyl as replacement of Pb in gasoline.

(*e*) Dyes, paints and pigments

(*f*) Pharmaceuticals and disinfectants

(*g*) Manganese mines: chronic inhalation of air-borne Mn in occupationally exposed subjects working in Mn mines, steel mills and some chemical industries.

SYSTEMIC EFFECTS [15,102,118,138,200,209]

In a case study of Mn poisoning in 15 miners in Chile, the following observations suggest nervous and reproductive systems to be more prone to the toxic effects of Mn vs. the other systems :

Symptoms	Incidence (%)
Neurological and psychosomatic disturbances	100
Disturbed libido	27
Difficulty in ejaculation	20

Other reports indicate inhalatory exposure to be more important for its adverse effects as compared to oral exposure.

1. ***Nervous system:*** Both experimental and clinical studies indicate brain to be the principal organ affected by Mn toxicity. Rats given Mn in drinking water (1 mg/ml) for 14-30 days exhibited hyperactivity, reduction in conditioned avoidance response and increase in the fighting scores. These behavioural changes were attributed to increased turnover of dopamine and nor-epinephrine. Initial manifestations are usually psychiatric symptoms *e.g.*, emotional instability, hallucinations and violent episodes. Manganese toxicity has been shown to produce learning disability in rats and increasing cholesterol biosynthesis. The clinical symptoms following chronic occupational exposure include akinesia, rigidity or mania which may progress to **Frank psychosis**, and a **syndrome resembling Parkinson's disease**. The latter occurs after many years of exposure and has been attributed to disturbances in dopamine, GABA, melanin and serotonin synthesis in the basal ganglia of brain. Pathological changes may be observed in the brain cortex, sub-cortical nuclei and

spinal cord. While most mental symptoms are alleviated after cessation of exposure, extra-pyramidal abnormalities are persistent and may last for years. Elevated hair Mn concentrations were reported in mentally-retarded children. **Sclerosis amyotrophic lateralis,** a disease reported from Japan, has been linked to high Mn content in soil and food chain. Reduced tissue Mn concentrations were found in some epileptic patients with frequent seizures and on therapy with anti-epileptic agents. Reduced Mn availability at the neuronal level (where Mn stabilizes membrane excitability) may affect epileptogenic lesions and increase likelihood of seizure activity. No links were discernible between the dementing disease and CSF Mn levels.

2. ***Liver:*** Manganese exerts hepatotoxic effect manifested by cirrhosis, fatty infiltration and perilobular necrosis. High liver and serum Mn levels are observed in acute viral hepatitis. The values return to near normal levels during subsiding phase of the disease after treatment. High hepatic (biopsy samples) and hair and low nail and urine concentrations of Mn were reported in Indian childhood cirrhosis. Serum Mn levels remained unaltered in ICC patients. Alcoholics and Fe-deficient subjects are more prone to the toxic effects of Mn. The metal was found to be a major component of biliary calculi.

3. ***Cardiovascular system:*** The lipotropic and enzymatic effects of Mn have been discussed under the sections on Role and Deficiency. Blood Mn concentrations are markedly elevated (to about twice the normal values) following coronary occlusion. The effect persists for several weeks. Blood Mn estimations are stated to be a better index of myocardial infarction vs. the conventional estimations. These aspects, however, need further validation.

5. ***Respiratory system:*** Environmental pollution and occupational exposure of workers through inhalatory route are known to cause Mn toxicity. It is manifested by pneumonia which can not be easily differentiated from non-occupational broncho- or lobular pneumonia. Reduced therapeutic efficacy and history of exposure may indicate Mn to be the etiology of respiratory symptoms.

6. ***Reproductive system:*** Both deficiency and excess of Mn has been linked to dysfunction of the reproductive system manifested by depressed libido, reduced desire and ability, difficulty in ejaculation, testicular damage, depressed sperm motility and migration, reduced fertility etc. Adenylcyclase (which is Mn^{2+} sensitive) activity is reported to have a positive correlation with sperm motility index. Elevated Mn levels, observed in the cervical mucus, during post-ovulatory phase make it unfavourable for sperm migration. No reports are available or any discernible changes in serum/tissue Mn levels during pregnancy.

7. ***Immune function:*** Experimental studies in mice and guinea pigs revealed decreased T cell-dependent antibody response, lymphokine production and host resistance to *Klebsiella pneumonia* and influenza virus infections following Mn administration. The latter, however, caused an increase in natural killer cell activity.

8. ***Haemopoietic system:*** Dietary intake of feeds containing > 2000 ppm Mn has been reported to inhibit hemoglobin synthesis by reducing Fe intake and its incorporation in the porphyrin ring causing sideroblastic anaemia.

9. ***Carcinogenic effects:*** Excess Mn may induce mutagenic and carcinogenic (direct or co-carcinogenic) effects. The former have been attributed in part to an effect on DNA polymerase. The mutagenic and carcinogenic actions, indicated by studies on microorganisms, need to be further confirmed in mammals.

10. ***Teratogenic effects:*** Teratogenic actions of Mn compounds have been reported in mice but not in human subjects.

MECHANISM OF TOXICITY [15,118]

(*a*) Disturbances in the metabolism of brain catecholamines.

(*b*) Inhibition of synthesis of dopamine, melanin and serotonin in the basal ganglia of brain.

(*c*) Enhanced lipid peroxidation (*per se* and in the form of lectins) by Mn interferes with ultrastructure and function of membranes.

(*d*) Caustic/corrosive actions by some Mn compounds *e.g.*, potassium permanganate which destroys the cells.

DIAGNOSTIC FEATURES [15,118]

History of exposure with:

(*i*) Symptoms particularly those affecting the extrapyramidal system causing Parkinson's disease type of syndrome.

(*ii*) Pathologic findings *e.g.*, corrosion of the mucus membranes and hemorrhages of the gastrointestinal tract with degenerative changes in liver and kidneys in cases of $KMnO_4$ poisoning.

TREATMENT [15,118]

- Chelation therapy: Though no universally-effective antidote is available, administration of Calcium EDTA in conjunction with supportive treatment may be given. It protects liver and the respiratory system but has no effect on CNS symptoms.
- Administration of L-3,4,-dihydroxy phenylalanine (L-DOPA) in early stages of the disease provides symptomatic relief.
- Special problems include management of intestinal perforations, respiratory distress, treatment of anurea etc.

MERCURY(Hg)

CATEGORY

- Non-essential accumulative trace element.

Distribution in Ecosystem [50,111,118]

AIR

	Hg ng/m^3
Remote Areas (Greenland)	NA
North America	2
Europe	1
India (Delhi)	95-136

WATER

	Hg µg/kg
River water	0.070
Sea water	0.002

SOIL

	Hg mg/kg
Surface soil	0.11

PLANT [118]

	Hg mg/kg (fresh weight)
Critical concentration at which no sensitivity develops in immature plants	1-3

PLANT FOODS [118]

	Hg µg/kg
Cereals, potatoes, vegetables fruits, tea coffee	4-40
Mushrooms	340

ANIMAL FOODS [50]

	Hg µg/kg
Milk	20
Beef	10-20
Chicken	40
Eggs	30
Shell fish	20
Organ meats (Liver)	upto 100

Methyl Hg is enriched in the aquatic food chain, concentration in predatory fish and whales may exceed 1 mg/kg.

Marine food contains Hg and Se in equimolar ratio with no harmful effects indicating their autoprotective effects in nature.

Methyl Hg is a neurotoxicant that bioaccumulates in the aquatic food chain and is present in all fish. Long-term low-level exposure (below commonly accepted 50-ppm threshold), has been reported to cause dose-dependent tremours. These effects were discernible on clinical examination. Interplay of other factors (*e.g.*, under-reported alcohol consumption cannot be ruled out.[16] Recent concerns of Hg and environmental toxins have clouded the clinical benefits of fish oil (Omega-3 fatty acids) which have been studied for more than 30 years. Some recent studies[11,136,175] highlighted its practical applications and utility in primary health care programmes.

MICROORGANISMS

Biomethylating microorganism : *Escherichia coli*

HUMAN BODY [93,118,158]

Whole Body Content

- Content in average adult man (60 kg) : 13 mg

Distribution

- Distributed in > 34 human tissues and body fluids with highest concentrations in kidney of exposed subjects.

	Hg µg/L
Blood	
Whole blood	< 5-20
Erythrocytes	7-50
Serum	12

	Hg µg/g (fresh weight)
■ **Tissues**	
Brain	0.1-0.3
Heart, Liver, Lungs, Skin	0.005-0.25
Kidneys	0.065-2.75

ROLE/ESSENTIALITY

- No physiological role is known for this metal.
- It is not required for the function of any enzyme or metabolic reaction.

DEFICIENCY

No deficiency syndrome has been recorded for any form of Hg.

METABOLISM [50,209]

Absorption

(*a*) ***Oral***

Absorption depends on the form of Hg; the values for dietary absorption in adult humans are as follows:

Form of Hg	Absorption %
Inorganic	7
Methyl	95

(*b*) ***Inhalation***

- This is the main route of exposure for Hg because of its monatomic nature, high vapour pressure, lipid solubility and high diffusibility.
- Approximately 80% of the inhaled Hg gets absorbed and retained in the body.

(*c*) ***Skin***

- Most forms of Hg can penetrate intact skin to some extent.
- Substantial systemic absorption occurs for alkyl mercurials. Topical dermal application of the latter may cause poisoning.

Distribution/Metabolism

Major part of methyl Hg in blood is found in erythrocytes (RBC : Plasma ratio is approx. 20). In contrast inorganic Hg shows equal distribution in RBC and Plasma. Mercury gets distributed to most tissues and body fluids including brain, placenta and foetus. Concentrations in kidney are the highest. Mercury vapours are rapidly oxidized in tissue to divalent ionic form Hg^{2+}. Organomercurials (*e.g.*, mercurial diuretics) undergo rapid transformation to inorganic Hg. Short chain alkyl Hg compounds (*e.g.*, methyl Hg) undergo slow transformation (< 1% per day) to inorganic form. Average half life for methyl Hg in man is about 70 days (range 46-120 days). Toxic properties of methyl Hg are partly due to the stability of C-Hg bond. The ratio of Hg content in erythrocytes to its plasma content depends on the form of Hg; it is highest for methyl Hg and lowest for inorganic Hg. Hair content is a useful index for assessing methyl Hg status; the concentration in hair is about 250 times higher than that in blood. Hg^{2+} have high affinity for SH groups and so these cations can cause widespread damage by altering functions of several bioproteins containing SH groups or disulphide bridges.

Excretion

The principal route of excretion is through feces but in cases of prolonged exposure, urinary excretion may marginally exceed fecal elimination. Excretion occurs through several routes: volatilization from lungs and skin, excretion in urine, sweat, milk, saliva, intestinal mucosa, bile, storage in and excretion via shed hair and nails. Urinary Hg concentrations have no correlation with blood Hg levels in populations heavily exposed to methyl Hg and so urine is a poor bioindicator for cases of methyl Hg poisoning.

INTAKE/REQUIREMENTS [118,208]

	Hg µg per day
■ Total dietary intake	
Children	2-6
Adults	2-140
■ Contribution from drinking water to dietary intake	2%

■ Fish and marine food account for 40% and vegetables and fruits for 20% of the total intake. Biotransformations in marine ecosystems may pose serious environmental problems.

■ No known minimum requirements.

GUIDELINES VALUES [118,209]

■ Occupational exposure limit (OEL) in air for 40-h work week	0.01-0.1 mg/m^3
OEL for pregnant females	Nil, no safe level

- Blood

Inorganic Hg	50 μg/l
Organic Hg	100 μg/l

- Urine <25 μg/l

  When urinary concentrations exceed 1-2 mg/L, Hg poisoning is suspected.

- Hair 50-125 μg/g
- Tolerable weekly intake per person

Total Hg	300 μg ; < 5 μg/kg per week
Methyl Hg	200 μg ; < 3.3 μg/kg per week

- Hazardous waste Category 4 (Govt. of India Manufacture, Storage and Import of Hazardous Chemical Rules 2000) if waste generates > 5 kg μg per year.

MEDICINAL USES [122,123,200,201]

Inorganic Hg compounds have been used as antiseptics, preservatives, parasiticidal and fungicidal agents. Mercury is not used internally in modern medicine. Calcined metal preparations (Ayurvedic and Unani) have, however, been attributed with many therapeutic properties. It is claimed that traditional calcination process, involving (*a*) incorporation of some herbal juices during the ashing process and (*b*) repeated ashing and grinding, detoxifies the metal and makes it therapeutically effective. Investigations on *Siddh Makardhwaja,* a reputed Ayurvedic preparation, revealed growth-promoting, memory-improving, glycogen-sparing (anti-fatigue) properties in rats and mice without discernible gross or subtle (on neurobehavioural parameters) toxicity. The preparation exhibited wide margin of safety (effective dose : 15 mg/kg po, maximum tolerated dose : > 16 g/kg po in rats and > 1g/kg ip in mice). Similarly, Ayurvedic *Kajjali Bhasma* and Unani *Kushta Sangraf* were shown to be tolerated at much higher doses than the known toxicities of these metals and their compounds. Toxic effects on various systems were, however, discernible when these traditional preparations were administered to rats and mice at high doses for 6 month. *Kushta Sangraf* exhibited some beneficial effects also *e.g.*, anticataleptic, glycogen sparing and favourable action on passive avoidance learning in experimental animals.

TOXICITY [13,50,77,101,200,209]

Sources of Exposure/Contamination

From extensive household and industrial uses in:

(*a*) Thermometers/barometers

(*b*) Mercury vapour lamps

(*c*) Dental amalgams

(*d*) Mirrors

(*e*) Chloralkali industry

(*f*) Electronic equipment

(*g*) Disinfectants/fungicides

(*h*) Synthetic silk industry

(*i*) Plastic industry

(*j*) Military detonators

(*k*) Medicinal uses for antiseptic, antibacterial skin ointments/lotions, laxative, diuretic purposes has mostly become obsolete in view of availability of better/safer agents.

(*l*) Most volatile metal. Chronic exposure by spills in poorly-ventilated laboratories with high Hg concentration in ambient air.

Toxic Dose

Acute lethal dose

Mercuric chloride	approx. 1-4g
Methyl mercury	10-60 mg/kg

MINAMATA DISEASE

This disease occurred on epidemic scale due to exposure to methyl mercury from consumption of :

(*a*) **Contaminated fish in Japan.** The first case was reported by Dr. Hosokowa in 1956 near Minamata Bay in Southern Japan. The contamination occurred due to effluent discharge from a chemical plant into the bay. The Hg load was so great that it killed fish and fish-eating birds which dropped into the sea with intense symptoms of violent whirl, dashing with a zig-zag course and collapse. Links between water pollution, consumption of contaminated fish and human disease could be established three years later in 1959 but unfortunately effluent dumping was not halted till 1968.

(*b*) **Contaminated bread in Iraq from organomercurial seed dressings/fungicides.** Over 60,000 people were affected with > 6000 hospital admissions and 200 deaths in 1971-72. Similar epidemics were later reported from other parts of the world: Canada, USA, New Zealand etc. **Primary risk groups**: Pregnant and nursing women owing to the susceptibility of the developing nervous system of the fetus and infant to the toxicity of methyl Hg.

Symptoms: Fatigue, loss of concentration and memory, low IQ values, headache, insomnia, drowsiness, numbness in limbs and face, paraesthesia, ataxia, treamours (fine trembling interrupted every few minutes by coarse shaking), dysarthria, constriction of visual field, cortical blindness, hearing defects, acute psychosis, slurred speech, imprecise handwriting with missing words, incoordinated gait etc. Abnormal muscle tone/deep tendon reflexes, higher incidence of abortions and still births etc. A typical comatose posture (arched neck, tightly-flexed arms, clenched fists and crossed legs, forced extension of limbs not possible) is observed. While the behavioural effects induced by methyl Hg are reversible, damage to fetal nervous system is usually permanent. Principal effect is elicited on the granular layer of cerebellum and visual cortex with neuronal loss and glial proliferation and the biochemical site of action is the SH group of enzymes.

PINK DISEASE

This Hg-induced syndrome occurs in children and is characterized by erythematous lesions in fingers, toes, cheeks, nose and buttocks. This imparts a pink look to the patient, hence the same.

SUDDEN DEATH

Cases of sudden death have been reported following i.v. use of mercurial diuretics in congestive heart failure. Death occurs within few minutes of injection due to ventricular fibrillation.

AMYOTROPHIC LATERAL SCLEROSIS

Exposure to Hg has been reported, in some cases, to be followed by a clinical picture resembling ALS.

SYSTEMIC EFFECTS [13,16,50,101,200,209]

1. ***Liver:*** Hepatic uptake of Hg^{2+} is independent of temperature and it does not involve SH-linked transsport or Ca channels. Within the liver cell, both inorganic and methyl forms react with intracellular thiols e.g., glutathione (GSH). While bulk of GSH (90%) is localized in cytosol, the mitochondrial GSH pool is critical for the hepatotoxic effects of Hg. Many traditional drugs (Ayurvedic/Unani) contain Hg compounds which may produce hepatotoxic effects. Substantial amounts of Hg accumulate in liver in Minamata disease.
2. ***Kidney:*** The metal accumulates in proximal tubules of kidneys, which is the critical organ for Hg, following ingestion of both inorganic and organic forms. Mercurial diuretics (mercaptomerin, mersalyl, mercurophylline etc.) elicit their effect by inhibiting tubular resorption of water. Diuresis is accompanied by urinary excretion of salts (Na, Cl) which contribute to the toxic effects of Hg. When mercurial diuretics are administered to pregnant females, the metal passes through the placenta and substantial amounts accumulate in fetal organs including kidneys. Post-natal exposure through breast milk of such mothers can also produce profound changes in proximal tubules of developing fetal kidneys.
3. ***Nervous system:*** Exposure to both inorganic and organic Hg compounds cause neurological damage and grave genetic defects. Axonal transport has been demonstrated in mice. The damage caused by alkyl Hg compounds is often irreversible. It is manifested by several neurological symptoms varying considerably in intensity from mild to serious which may be fatal. The classical example of such exposure is Minamata disease (please see page 150). In a study on 53 patients with positive methyl Hg poisoning, the frequency (%) of neurological signs and symptoms was reported as follows:

Symptom	Frequency (%)
Cerebral disturbances	95
Sensory impairment	65
Visual disturbance	60
Speech disturbances	75
Mental abnormality	50
Pyramidal tract lesions	38
Hearing defects	19
Involuntary movements	31
Cranial nerves involvement (other than optic)	19
Autonomic disorders	19
Encephalopathy	32

4. ***Cardiovascular system:*** The metal may cause arrhythmias, atrioventricular dissociation, extrasystoles, ventricular tachycardia, fibrillation and cardiovascular collapse (Please see sudden death following use of mercurial diuretics under Toxicity section, page 151). Chronic exposure in drinking water or food leads to elevated BP in animals and man.
5. ***Respiratory system:*** Acute inhalation of inorganic Hg is manifested by irritant/inflammatory symptoms: cough, bronchitis, dyspnoea, chest pain and pneumonia. Chronic exposure to organic Hg compounds may cause nasal catarrh and epistaxis.
6. ***Skin:*** Inorganic and organic Hg compounds elicit antiseptic, parasiticidal and fungicidal properties. The alkyl and alkoxy compounds cause local irritation and systemic poisoning when absorbed hypersensitivity skin reactions (erythema, eruptions) may occur following therapeutic use of mercurial diuretics. The effect may be local or generalized (Please see Pink disease, page 151).
7. ***Reproductive system:*** Toxic effects are manifested in both males (deformation in seminiferous tubules and Leydig cells) and females (intrauterine death, fetal resorptions, still births). Considerable inter-species variations for such effects have been reported. Human effects came to light during epidemics in Japan and Iraq (page, 150, 154).
8. ***Immune function:*** Nephrotoxic effects are immunologically mediated. Studies in experimental animals revealed the following effects on different components of immune function:

DECREASE	INCREASE
(*a*) Weight of thymus gland and spleen (*b*) T cell-dependent antibody response	(*a*) ß-lymphocyte proliferation (*b*) Positive response to anti-nuclear antibodies
(*c*) T-lymphocyte proliferation	(*c*) Positive response to contact-sensitization tests.
(*d*) Concanavalin A activity	(*d*) Mortality from virus infection.
(*e*) Both primary and secondary immune responses impaired by methyl Hg.	(*e*) Methyl Hg showed stimulatory effect on mixed lymphocyte cultures in some studies.

Recently an inorganic Hg compound thimerosal (Et Hg) was shown to elicit initial immunosuppressive effects similar to those of MeHg leads in genetically susceptible mice to a second phase with strong immunostimulation and autoimmunity, which is T-cell dependent, H_2-linked and may at least partly be due to inorganic Hg derived from the metabolism of Et Hg.[83]

9. ***Carcinogenic effects:*** The metal is reported to possess anti-mitotic and cytotoxic properties and it was shown to induce chromosomal aberrations, renal tumours and sarcomas in rodents. Evidence for association of Hg with human cancer is inadequate.

10. ***Teratogenic effects:*** Methyl Hg crosses the placental barrier and since its post-natal excretion is very slow, high levels (19-fold higher vs. adults) of Hg are observed in suckling rats. While inorganic Hg does not readily cross the placental barrier, infants can acquire significant amounts from breast milk. Organic mercurials were shown to elicit embryotoxic and teratogenic effects in experimental animals (mice, rats, rabbits), domestic animals and humans. The effects include:

(*a*) Intra-uterine death

(*b*) Fetal resorptions

(*c*) Still births

(*d*) Cleft palate

(*e*) Facial malformations

(*f*) Abnormal skull and teeth

(*g*) Missing limbs

(*h*) Encephalopathy

(*i*) Encephalocele

(*j*) Hydrocephalus

(*k*) Cataract

(*l*) Growth retardation

(*m*) Ataxia

(*n*) Cerebral palsy

(*o*) Neuro-behavioural deficit

It is believed that ingestion of 1 kg fish contaminated with methyl Hg (even within legal limits) may produce significant behavioural deficits in new born infants. The biochemical markers for methyl Hg are elevated concentrations of orinthine decarboxylase in fetal brain and kidneys. Pre-natal and post-natal exposure is manifested by pathological changes in developing nervous system.

Epidemiological studies from Japan and Iraq indicated that while the deliveries were apparently normal in exposed women, later observations revealed: (*a*) depressed physical and mental development, (*b*) decreased alertness and I.Q. (*c*) ataxia and cerebral palsy, (*d*) abnormalities of skull and teeth in infants. The damage to fetal nervous system is usually permanent. Some degree of ataxia was discernible in surviving offsprings even after 30 years of Minamata epidemic.

MECHANISMS OF TOXICITY [15,50,77,118]

(*a*) Affinity for thiol groups.

(*b*) Neurotoxic effects of methyl Hg and inorganic Hg are distinctly different.

Inorganic Hg	*Methyl Hg*
(*i*) Mainly sensori-motor effects by Hg vapour	(*i*) Mainly neuropsychiatric effects
(*ii*) More potent inhibitor of brain muscarinic receptors (Potency 100 times more vs. methyl Hg)	(*ii*) Mild effect on brain muscarinic receptors.

(*c*) Enhancement of lipid peroxidation

(*d*) Alterations in intracellular Ca^{2+}

(*e*) Impairment of primary and secondary immune response.

DIAGNOSTIC FEATURES [15,50,77,118]

Diagnosis of Hg poisoning is based on:

1. ***History:*** Hg exposure form (elemental, inorganic, organic), dose, route etc.
2. ***Clinical presentation:*** Among the signs and symptoms, described under systemic effects, generalized erythema (Pink disease), neuro-behavioural and renal effects are diagnostic. The

following signs and symptoms are also important in cases of Hg poisoning: metallic taste, gingivitis, dark lines on gums (HgS), stomatitis, polyuria progressing to oliguria and then anuria, chest pain, skin reactions etc.

3. *Laboratory investigations:*

3.1 *Blood examination:*

Hg level > 4 μg/dl

RBC : Plasma Hg concentration ratio indicates type of poisoning. Higher ratio is indicative for methyl Hg.

3.2 *Urine examination:*

– Hg concentrations in normal urine should be < 25 μg/l.

– Elemental Hg in urine exhibits a linear relationship with plasma Hg concentrations.

– Urinary values 500 μg/l are associated with treamours.

– Urine is a poor indicator for methyl Hg which is mainly excreted in feces.

3.3 *Hair examination:*

– Hair are rich in SH groups and so contain 250 times more Hg vs. blood.

– Analysis for Hg in different segments of hair may give a clue to the duration of exposure (Growth rate: 20 cm per year).

TREATMENT OF MERCURY POISONING [15,77,118]

ELEMENTAL Hg (VAPOUR)	INORGANIC Hg SALTS	ORGANIC Hg COMPOUNDS
■ Immediate termination of exposure	■ Prompt fluid therapy ■ Maintaining electrolyte balance	■ Mobilization of methyl Hg from body is difficult because transport from tissues to blood is rapid but from blood to urine is slow.
■ Close monitoring of pulmonary status.	■ Monitoring hematological status	Enteropathic recirculation and redistribution occurs.
■ Respiratory support if necessary	■ Removal of unabsorbed Hg and preventing its further absorption: - Magnesium cathartic - Gastric lavage - Activated charcoal - Emesis if patient is alert and awake.	■ Hemodialysis, hemoperfusion and peritoneal dialysis remove negligible amounts of Hg as it is concentrated in RBCs and little is available unbound in plasma. ■ Hemodialysis with infusion of cysteine or N-acetyl penicillamine is useful.

- **Chelation therapy** is initiated after the above mentioned measures and continued depending upon the clinical condition of the patient.
- **Dimercaprol** is recommended in inorganic Hg poisoning but its use and efficacy in organic and elemental Hg poisoning is questionable. If administered alone, it gets re-distributed throughout the body. Its complex with Hg causes renal damage.
- **Penicillamine** It has relatively poor efficacy and so large doses are required. It is more suitable for low exposure levels and asymptomatic cases. D-penicillamine reverses SH-binding of Hg in the blood and chelates the metal. Hemodialysis with N-acetyl penicillamine is useful. The use of this chelating agent is contraindicated in penicillin-sensitive patients.
- ***Unithiol*** and ***Polythiol*** resins can be used.
- **Newer chelating agents** DMSA and DMPS
- **Supportive therapy** Using polysaccharides, lipotropic agents, vitamin B_{12} and folic acid.

MOLYBDENUM(Mo)

CATEGORY

Essential trace element.

DISTRIBUTION IN ECOSYSTEM [118]

WATER	Mo $\mu g/m^3$
River water	1
Sea water	10
SOIL	
Calcareous soils of Western USA, Canada	6 ppm
Acid soils of Eastern USA	0.5 ppm
Content is generally low in acid and freely drained soils and high in humus soils with impeded drainage.	

PLANTS/PLANT FOODS [118,209]

- Uptake of Mo increases with increase in pH of soil.
- Biological accumulation index/plant: soil ratio: 0.1 to 1.0

■ **Edible Plants**

	Mo mg/kg fresh weight
Cereals	2.55
Vegetables	0.07-1.0
Fruits	0.002 - 0.16
Mushrooms	0.032
Tea	0.13

■ Mo-dependent enzymes are involved in nitrogen fixation.

ANIMAL FOODS [15]

Mo content in animal products is low.

		Mo μg/kg (fresh weight)
Milk and dairy products	:	70 (50-110)
Meat	:	20-50
Eggs	:	90
Sea foods	:	20-100
Liver and organ meats	:	1000-3000

HUMAN BODY [15,93,158]

Whole Body Content

■ 0.1 ppm

■ Content in average adult man (60 kg) : 9.3 mg

Distribution

Presence of Mo has been reported in at least 40 human tissues and body fluids including blood, brain, liver, kidneys, lungs, spleen, muscles etc. It is a constituent of following metalloenzymes:

(*i*) Nitrogenase

(*ii*) Xanthine dehydrogenase/oxidase

(*iii*) Nitrate reductase

(*iv*) Aldehyde oxidase

(*v*) Sulphite oxidase

It is also present in flavoproteins.

ROLE/ESSENTIALITY [118,200,209]

All known functions of Mo are due to molybdenoenzymes.

(*a*) It is involved in N fixation by microorganisms in higher plants leading to protein synthesis. Vegetarian food is, therefore, rich in Mo and the content in animal origin food is low. Fertilizers containing Mo increase crop yield.

(*b*) Mo participates in essential redox reactions *in vivo*. Three principle enzymes viz. xanthine dehydrogenase, aldehyde oxidase and sulphite oxidase share a common cofactor viz. molybdopterin. It is a substituted protein to which Mo is bound by two S atoms. These enzymes also contain Fe, S and Flavin. Xanthine dehydrogenase converts tissue purines to uric acid. If this reaction occurs with O, free radicals are generated which cause tissue damage. Sulphite oxidase is involved in conversion of sulfite (derived from S containing amino acids cystine and methionine) into inorganic sulphate. Absence results in toxic accumulation of sulphite in critical organs/tissues.

(*c*) Role in maturation of hematological cells. In cases of hemochromatosis, high hepatic Mo concentrations have been reported.

(*d*) Role in pregnancy and early stages of development.

(*e*) Interactions occur with several elements *e.g.*, Cu, F, Fe, S, Wo. Antagonism to Cu has been reported. Low Mo levels are observed in cases of Fe-deficiency anaemia secondary to malignant tumours.

(*f*) Relationship with Keshan's disease has been suggested but not confirmed. High Mo levels have been reported in many diseases *e.g.*, rheumatoid arthritis, Laennec's cirrhosis, hemochromatosis, uremia etc.

DEFICIENCY [118,200,209]

Dietary deficiency is rare. Deficiency may occur in patients on prolonged parenteral nutrition.

Experimental/Farm Animals

Experimental deficiency can be induced in animals by feeding high levels of Tungsten (45-94 mg/kg) in diet. Deficiency of molybdopterin and Mo containing enzymes causes adverse effects.

Deficiency of Xanthine dehydrogenase following low Mo and protein intake or in cases of hepatoma may be clinically manifested by renal calculi and mild myopathy due to xanthine deposition in muscles. Deficiency of sulphite oxidase due to a genetic defect may be manifested by neurological symptoms and high urinary output of sulphite in mammals. Deficiency in goats has been reported to exert an inhibitory effect on reproductive function causing reduced fertility and fetal survival.

Human studies

(*a*) Patients on prolonged total parenteral nutrition exhibited following symptoms:

- Irritability
- Tonic/clonic seizures
- Tachycardia
- Tachypnoea
- Night blindness/ Discoloured lenses
- Coma

The clinical symptoms were associated with low blood and liver molybdopterin, sulfite oxidase, xanthine and dehydrogenase levels and enhanced excretion of sulphite, thiosulphate, s-sulphocystein, xanthine and hypoxanthine. The symptoms were reversed by supplementation with ammonium molybdate (300-500 μg/day). Beneficial effect was also observed following reduced intake of proteins and S containing amino acids. Oral molybdate had no effect in clinical condition and urinary excretion because of deficiency of active cofactor. According to some reports parenteral infusion with 500 μg ammonium molybdate, lead to increased uric acid concentrations in plasma and urine. The adverse effects were increased by infusion of sulfite.

(*b*) Low Mo content in drinking water has been linked to higher incidence of oesophageal cancer. Evidence for anticarcinogenic effects of Mo is, however, incomplete.

(*c*) Molybdenum accumulates in teeth. It remains to be seen whether depleted states cause dental caries.

(*d*) Low Mo content has been reported in cereals and water in areas affected with Keshan's disease. Concurrent deficiency of Mo with Se has been suggested for this disease. Fertilizers containing Mo reduce the incidence of Keshan's disease.

METABOLISM [42]

Absorption

Gastrointestinal absorption depends on the form in which Mo is ingested: Mo (IV) sulfide: 5% only; most other Mo compounds: 50-80%, more absorption for soluble compounds. The absorption is inhibited by luminal concentration of SO_4 anion.

Distribution/Metabolism

Residence time in gastrointestinal tract may extend upto 14 days. Approximately 40% of ingested Mo appears in all major organs/tissues. The distribution is reported in > 40 human tissues and body fluids. Sulfates present as such or generated from breakdown of S containing amino acids, act as Mo antagonist and inhibit utilization of this element.

Excretion

Excretion is almost complete and occurs mostly through urine.

INTAKE/REQUIREMENTS [209]

Wide variations are observed in reported values.

	Mo µg/day
Median intake (range)	120 (60-520)
Requirements	2.0

GUIDELINE VALUES [118,209]

	Mo µg/kg body weight
Upper limits for safe human intake	140-200
	Mo mg/m³ of air
Occupational exposure level	5.0

MEDICINAL USES

1. Use in deficiency states described above.
2. Tetrathiomolybdate is useful in cases of Cu toxicity and as an alternative to penicillamine in Wilsons's disease.

TOXICITY [15,118,195,200,209]

Sources of Exposure

1. Foundary workers
2. Uranium mines
3. Molybdenum milling
4. Oil refining and coal power plants
5. Flora enrichment with Mo fertilizers etc.

Toxicity in Animals and Man

Increased air concentrations may cause toxicity, links have been reported with incidence of mortality from bronchitis, pneumonia and lung cancer. There is considerable species variation for Mo toxicity. **Molybdenosis** is also called **Teart syndrome** or **Peat scours** in farm animals. Calves given Mo (50 ppm) in drinking water show depleted tissue Cu uptake and increased serum ceruloplasmin levels with neuropsychiatric manifestations. Toxicity was also observed when rats were given Mo 2-6 mg/kg/day as Ammonium thiomolybdate in diet.

Toxicity with Mo in human beings is not a major problem. It is linked to induction of Cu deficiency and/or inadequate utilization of Cu and defect in osteogenesis. The symptoms include :

(*a*) Anorexia, diarrhoea

(*b*) Bronchitis, pneumonia, high incidence of lung cancer

(*c*) Elevated uric acid levels.

(*d*) Fatigue

(*e*) Headache

(*f*) Pain in joints

(*g*) Bone deformities

(*h*) Spontaneous fractures

(*i*) Tremours in hands

(*j*) CNS disturbances

(*k*) Fluorosis and endemic gout

(*l*) Depigmentation of hair/wool

(*m*) Loss of hair etc.

MECHANISM OF TOXICITY [15]

Cu antagonism

DIAGNOSTIC FEATURES [15]

(*a*) Increased serum Mo and ceruloplasmin levels.

(*b*) Symptoms specially frequent fractures, gout and neuropsychiatric manifestations.

TREATMENT [15]

(*a*) Chelating Agents : Unithiol

Sodium sulphate

(*b*) Cu-enriched diet : 8-10 ppm of Cu in diet has been shown to protect cattle, sheep against 5-6 ppm Mo.

(*c*) Methionine.

NEODYMIUM (Nd)

CATEGORY

Non-essential accumulative trace element.

DISTRIBUTION IN ECOSYSTEMS [118]

Earth's crust	28 ppm

HUMAN BODY [93,193]

Presence of Nd has been shown in whole blood, serum, lungs, lymph nodes, testes and tooth enamel.

TOXICITY [118]

Intravenous injection of Nd nitrate was shown to be highly toxic to female rats (male rats were less susceptible).

NEON (Ne)

CATEGORY

Inert gas. Not reported in human body.

NICKEL (Ni)

CATEGORY

Possibly essential ultra-trace element.

As late as in 1971, Williams[131] stated that though this element is abundant in nature, it is not found *in vivo* because it is strongly held in minerals and so can not enter plants and then our bodies. With advancement of knowledge, now not only it is known to be present in human body, it has also been attributed with some essential functions.

DISTRIBUTION IN ECOSYSTEM TY [15,111]

AIR

	Ni ng/m³
North America	100
Europe	25
North India (wide range of values reported)	12-321

WATER

	Ni mg/m³
Sea water	0.6
Fresh water	0.5
Drinking water*	2-5 μg/L

* Typical tap water concentrations. Assuming a consumption of 2 litres water per day, the intake through drinking water alone will be 4-10 μg/day. Exceptionally levels in drinking water may reach upto 500 μg/L. No guideline value has been set.

SOIL

Ni content	**mg/kgf**
Mean (range)	20 (5-35)

PLANT FOODS [15,118,133]

	mg/kgf
Cereals, potatoes, vegetables, fruits	0.05-0.35
Tea	5.25
Coffee	0.77

Examination of Ni content in selected herbs, herbal fruit teas and their infusions revealed that the amount of Ni present in these is not harmful to human health.[34,147]

ANIMAL FOODS [15,118,132]

Milk	10-30 μg/L
Meats	1-13 μg/kgf
Organ meats *e.g.*, Bovine liver	70-180 μg/kgf

HUMAN BODY [93,158]

Whole Body Content

- 1.0×10^{20} atoms in the body
- 1.0×10^{6} atoms in each cell
- 0.1 ppm
- Content in an average adult man (60 kg) : approx. 10 mg

Distribution

- Distributed in > 43 tissues/body fluids including blood, brain, liver, kidneys, lungs, skeleton etc.

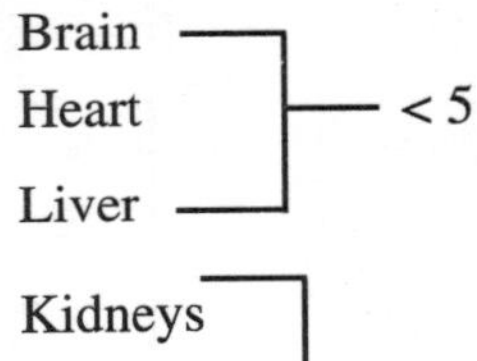

		Ni µg/L Mean (range)
■ Blood	RBC	83 (48-106)
	Plasma	54 (10-66)
		Ni µg/g ash
■ Tissues	Brain, Heart, Liver	< 5
	Kidneys, Lungs	< 5-24
	Skin	47

ROLE [3,59,118,120,200]

- Biochemical and physiological functions are not well understood at present.
- Probably plays a role in:
  - (*a*) Structure of membranes
  - (*b*) Lipid metabolism/glucose tolerance
  - (*c*) Regulation of prolactin
  - (*d*) Structural organization of DNA and RNA
  - (*e*) Enzymatic functions: deoxyribonuclease, acetyl co-enzyme A synthetase, phosphoglucomutase etc.
  - (*f*) Constituent of urease (not present in man). Its absence inhibits N fixation in soil.

DEFICIENCY [3,59,118,120,200,203]

- Deficiency syndrome described in many species of laboratory and farm animals *e.g.*, rat, minipig, chick, cow, goat, sheep etc.
- *Symptoms include:*
  - (*i*) growth retardation
  - (*ii*) ultrastructural abnormalities in liver.
  - (*iii*) altered Fe metabolism with impaired Fe utilization, depressed hematopoiesis, reduced hemoglobin and RBC count.
  - (*iv*) unthriftiness, rough skin and uneven hair.
  - (*v*) delayed estrus and perinatal mortality.
  - (*vi*) human deficiency not reported but reduced Ni levels are observed in patients with cirrhosis of liver and uremia.
  - (*vii*) deficiency syndrome observed in animals and claimed reversal by Ni supplementation are sometimes questioned and thought to be manifestations of pharmacological actions of Ni.

METABOLISM [3,15,118,209]

Absorption

- ***Oral:*** Less than 10% of ingested Ni is absorbed. The absorption is more during Fe deficiency state, pregnancy and lactation. Transfer across membranes is not by simple diffusion. It is an energy driven process linked to Fe transport system. Principal site of absorption is proximal part of the small intestines. Presence of food and beverages in the gastro-intestinal tract inhibits the rate of absorption.
- ***Inhalation:*** Approximately 35% of inhaled Ni is rapidly absorbed from lungs.
- ***Skin:*** Absorption also occurs through intact skin.

DISTRIBUTION/METABOLISM

- Transport of Ni^{2+} is mediated through bound forms. Binding occurs with albumin and unfiltrable ligands *e.g.*, amino-acids, histidine and cysteine and small polypeptides.
- ***Nickeloplasmin:*** an α-macroglobulin is a major Ni-binding protein but it does not play a significant role in extracellular transport. This is because the Ni, so bound, is not readily exchangeable with exogenous Ni. Binding also occurs with RNA.

- It crosses blood brain barrier but brain Ni concentrations are less vs. those in other tissues/organs. Nickel carbonyl is lipid soluble and one of the most toxic Ni compound.
- Interactions have been reported with prolactin and several elements *e.g.*, Ca, Cr, Cu, Co, I, Fe, Mg, Mn, Mo, P, K, Na, Zn etc.
- It also crosses the placental barrier and reaches fetus.

Excretion

- As most of the ingested Ni (90%) remains unabsorbed, the major route of excretion is through feces.
- Urinary excretion is small. It occurs in the form of low molecular weight complexes with histidine and aspartic acid.
- Significant amount is excreted through sweat.
- Other routes of excretion include exhaled air, milk and hair.

INTAKE/REQUIREMENTS [118,209]

- Average intake values are quite varied : < 70 to > 200 μg/day. The dietary intake varies at different places (UK : 140-145, USA : 69-112, Denmark : 130 μg/day) and with type of food consumed: plant (high Ni) or animal (low Ni) origin food and also with processing/refining.
- Most monogastric animals have a Ni requirement of < 200 μg/kg of diet. Precise human requirement has not been worked out. From extrapolation of animal data, basic requirement for an average adult is estimated to be < 100 μg per day. A dietary intake 300 - 900 μg/day should fulfil this requirement.
- Serum values > 1 μg/L Ni are reported to indicate chronic excessive intake of Ni.

GUIDELINE VALUES [118,209]

■ Occupational exposure limit (OEL) in air for 40-h work week	0.1- 1.0 mg/m^3
■ Blood Ni	0.05-1.05 μg/l
■ Urine Ni	0.5-6.1 μg/l
■ Maximum permissible concentration in waste water for biological treatment	1 mg/l

TOXICITY 15,50,118,120,153,209

Sources of Exposure/Contamination

From industrial and household usage in:

(*a*) Alloys for corrosion-resistant equipment

(*b*) Cooking utensils

(*c*) Coinage

(*d*) Electroplating

(*e*) Paints and pigments

(*f*) Hooks, fasteners, artificial jewellery, hair pins, cosmetics, shampoos etc.

(*g*) Heating elements

(*h*) Batteries

(*i*) Gas turbines, jet engines

(*j*) Ni carbonyl, which is extensively used in the manufacture of metallic Ni, is the most toxic compound of this metal

(*k*) High quality stainless steel utensils are considered safe

(*l*) Orthodontics/Dental amalgams

(*m*) Welding

SYSTEMIC EFFECTS 15,50,118,200,209

1. ***Liver:*** High hepatic and low serum Ni levels have been observed in patients with fatty and non-fatty cirrhosis.

2. ***Kidney:*** Dystrophic changes are observed in kidneys of animals intoxicated with Ni. Renal parenchyma, distal tubular lining of cells and mitochondria from renal tissue of such animals show elevated Ni concentrations. Patients with diffuse glomerulonephritis exhibit hypernickelemia and reduced concentrations of Ni in urine. Low serum Ni levels are usually observed in uremic patients.

3. ***Central nervous system:*** Marked hypothermia and diminution of metabolic rate has been reported mice given an i.p. injection of $NiCl_2$. Cerebral hemorrhages are observed in fatal cases of nickel carbonyl poisoning.

4. ***Cardiovascular system:*** Nickeloplasmin, a Ni-containing macroglobulin, is present in rabbit and human serum. While its precise physiological function is not known, an increase in serum Ni has been reported in cases of acute stroke and myocardial infarction. Patients with acute myocardial ischemia without infarctions, acute trauma with fractured bones, acute delirium tremens and muscular dystrophy, exhibited normal serum Ni concentrations. Therefore, monitoring of changes in serum Ni concentrations during the first 7 days may have a diagnostic potential in myocardial infarction. Toxicity due to Ni may be manifested in cardio-pulmonary insufficiency, electro-cardiographic abnormalities and dystrophic changes in the cardiac muscle. Conflicting reports are available for effects on the hemopoietic system in both animals and man. Oral exposure in rats has been reported to reduce hemoglobin, hematocrit and packed cell volume. Opposite results were shown following inhalatory exposure for 21 days in female rats. Erythrocytosis resulted following intratracheal injection. Probably both gender and route of exposure influence the action. Chronic intoxication with Ni carbonyl results in phased alteration of the blood picture. During the first year of contact, stimulation of erythropoiesis and after five years of exposure a tendency to leucopenia is noted. Reduction in the hemoglobin content and erythrocyte count have also been observed in Ni toxicity.

5. ***Respiratory system:*** Lung is the primary target organ for Ni toxicity. The signs and symptoms include dyspnoea, cough, intense chest pain, cyanosis and broncho-alveolar hyperplasia. Industrial exposure may cause lung cancer. Occupationally exposed electroplating and electrolytic refinery workers (who inhale vapours of water soluble Ni salts) develop chronic respiratory diseases *e.g.*, asthma, bronchitis, rhinitis, sinusitis, nasal polyps, pneumoconiosis and perforation of nasal septum. Inhalation of Ni carbonyl produces malaise, weakness, tachycardia and shortness of breath initially which may lead to pulmonary edema, respiratory failure and death.

6. ***Skin:*** Salts of Ni constitute an important cause of contact dermatitis and eczema. Allergic contact dermatitis has been reported in sensitive female populations from hair pins, imitation jewellery, brassier hooks and other metal fastenings on clothing. Ear piercing in combination with Ni jewellery is a primary cause of Ni sensitization. Dermatitis has also been observed in the palms of hair dressers from frequent use of Ni-containing shampoos. Cross reactivity with other metals *e.g.*, Cr is common. Dermatitis may be aggravated by oral intake of Ni containing foods *e.g.*, chocolates and nuts as also by some drugs *e.g.*, disulfiram and indomethacin. European battery of standard patch tests includes nickel sulphate (5% solution). An oral dose of as low as 0.6 mg given with water to fasting subjects, has been reported to produce skin reactions in some Ni-sensitive individuals. It is interesting to note that experimental Ni deficiency in chicken, rats and swine causes skin discolouration, dermatitis and loss of hair and these symptoms are corrected by dietary Ni supplementation.

7. ***Reproductive system:*** Nickel plays a role in the regulation of prolactin. Depressed reproductive performance has been observed in Ni-deficient animals which is normalised on Ni supplementation. Experimental toxicity in rats adversely affects male reproductive function by causing reduced testosterone levels, increased chromatolysis, desquamation in the spermatogenic epithelium, testicular atrophy, shrinkage of seminiferous tubules, impaired spermatogenesis, reduced sperm motility and disintegration of spermatozoa. Foetal resorptions and embryonic mortality were observed in female rats.

8. ***Immune function:*** Nickel is a potent skin sensitizer with reported prevalence of Ni sensitivity of 8-14% in women and 1% in men. Immunotoxicity and allergic reactions due to this metal are frequently observed following external exposure to its alloys (jewellery, coinage) or following oral intake or inhalation. Animal studies revealed pulmonary alveolar macrophages to be the primary targets of the immunotoxic effects of Ni. Acute or chronic exposure of mice, guinea pigs and rabbits was shown to suppress: (*a*) macrophage function, (*b*) antibody response to T cell-dependent antigens, (*c*) response of lymphocytes to T and B cell mitogens, (*d*) delayed hypersensitivity reactions and (*e*) systemic natural killer cell function. Exposure to Ni has been shown to generate Ni-specific T-lymphocytes probably mediated by interaction of Ni with major histocompatible class II peptide complex. Intra-tracheal administration of Ni, however, enhanced natural killer cell activity in bronchial lavage cells of monkeys. Decreased phagocytic activity with no effect on the number of primary antibody forming cells was also noted in this study. The clinical relevance of these reports remains to be elucidated.

9. ***Carcinogenic and Genotoxic effects:*** Experimental and epidemiological evidence indicates Ni to be mutagenic and carcinogenic in both animal models and man. High intracellular concentration of Ni appears to damage selectively the genetically-inactive heterochromatin. The damage may involve cross-linking of oxidized aminoacids to DNA. Administration of soluble salts in drinking water promotes the carcinogenic action of nitrosamine in rats. The metal has been linked to the incidence of malignant tumours of nasal cavity, larynx, sinuses and lungs following occupational exposure of Ni refinery workers to Ni dust and Ni carbonyl vapours. The average latent period was reported to be 22 years (range: 6-30 years). A correlation was also shown between Ni concentrations in town water supplies in Iowa (USA) and the incidence of lung and bladder cancers. Higher amounts of Ni were reported in food chain in areas with high incidence of cancer vs. other rural areas in Poland.

10. ***Teratogenic effect:*** Experimental evidence exists for teratogenic and embryotoxic effects of Ni compounds in mice, rats and hamsters. The metal elicits its adverse actions in the developing organism at relatively small doses in the early stages of pregnancy. Nickel chloride administered to pregnant rats caused foetal resorptions, increased embryonic

mortality and foetal malformations. Ocular abnormalities *e.g.*, anophthalmia and microphthalmia in rat pups and exencephaly and cystic lungs in hamster pups were reported following exposure to nickel carbonyl. Human placenta is permeable to Ni compounds. This is evident from analysis of Ni in human embryos which show peak accumulation between 12 to 19 weeks of pregnancy. Reports regarding its effects on the new-born are not available.

MECHANISM OF TOXICITY [3,15,118]

(*a*) Nickel carbonyl inhibits ATPase and RNA polymerase activities in target tissues.

(*b*) Peroxidative degradation of membrane lipids.

(*c*) Inhibition of natural killer cell activity, T cell mediated immune response and macrophage function.

(*d*) Allergenic and carcinogenic actions.

DIAGNOSTIC FEATURES [15,118]

(*i*) Symptoms particularly allergenic/carcinogenic effects on skin and respiratory system.

(*ii*) Patch tests : Ni sulphate (5%) in petroleum vehicle.

(*iii*) Dimethylglyoxime spot test is used to detect metals which leach more than 10 µg of Ni.

TREATMENT [15,118]

- Chelation therapy using BAL or unithiol
- Lanolin castor ointment protects the skin against harmful effects of Ni.
- Symptomatic treatment include:

  (*i*) Anti-inflammatory agents, (*ii*) Antibiotics, (*iii*) Blood letting, (*iv*) Diuretics etc. These measures give relief from inflammatory states of respiratory mucosa and pulmonary oedema.

NIOBIUM (Nb)

CATEGORY

Non-essential accumulative ultra-trace element.

DISTRIBUTION IN ECOSYSTEMS [118]

Earth's crust	24 ppm
Land plants	0.4-1.0 mg/kg dry weight.

HUMAN BODY [93,193]

Whole body content in average adult man (60 kg): 112 mg

It is widely distributed, presence has been reported in about 20 human tissues and body fluids including all vital organs, blood, bones, tooth enamel and hair.

ROLE/ESSENTIALITY

No nutritional/physiological role or deficiency syndrome has been attributed to this element.

METABOLISM [118]

Oral absorption is very poor. Studies in adult rats revealed it to be approximately 1% of the administered dose. Absorption was much higher in suckling rats. Inhalatory exposure may lead to substantial absorption (60%). Tracer studies revealed higher retention in lungs. Excretion occurs via urine and feces.

GUIDELINE VALUE [118]

Occupational Exposure Limit for Nb hydride in air : 6 mg/m^3

TOXICITY [118]

Sources of Exposure/Contamination

(*a*) Ferroniobium used to alloy Cu and stainless steel, on-ferrous metals, and metals used in arc welding rods.

(*b*) Alloys used in pipeline construction.

(c) Ti-Al-Nb alloys in biocompatible high strength surgical implants.

(*d*) Dentistry

(*e*) Superconductors

(*f*) Ceremics etc.

ANIMALS

Respiratory paralysis in cats (lethal). LD_{50}: rats 14 mg/kg, mice 21 mg/kg i.p. No mutagenic effects reported.

MAN

No information available.

NITROGEN (N)

CATEGORY

Essential bulk element. Constituent of the basic structure of human body.

HUMAN BODY [93,118,210,211]

Whole Body Content

- 13.5 million atoms per billion atoms.
- 2.3% of total weight of protoplasm
- 34 g/kg of fat-free tissues.
- 26,000 ppm
- Total content in average adult man (60 kg): approx. 1.8 kg

Distribution

- Ingredient of all organic matter.
- Essential constituent of proteins.
- Present in all tissues and body fluids.

ROLE [182]

- Reflects protein status of the body.
- N balance studies are carried out to determine protein status.
- A positive N balance is desirable in adults. Negative N balance occurs in disease states, fever, toxaemia, stress and surgery.

REQUIREMENT

16 g/day

OSMIUM (Os)

CATEGORY

Non-essential accumulative ultra-trace element.

HUMAN BODY [93,193]

Presence has been reported in blood and dentine of teeth.

GUIDELINE VALUES [118]

Occupational Exposure Limit for Os oxide in air (MAK Germany) : 0.2 μg/m^3

Upper limit in waste water (Germany) : 3 mg/L

TOXICITY [118]

For physiological incompatibility to living cells, Os is considered in close proximity to Pb. Action of Os oxide on mucus membranes can lead to dimming of cornea with reversible impairment of vision. Handling Os tetra oxide can lead to toxic effects.

OXYGEN (O)

CATEGORY

Essential bulk element. Constituent of the basic structure of human body.

HUMAN BODY [15,158,210,211]

Whole Body Content

- 255 million atoms per billion atoms.
- 65% of total weight of protoplasm
- 10,000 ppm
- Total content in average adult man (60 kg): 43 kg

Distribution

- Ingredient of all organic matter.
- Present in all tissues and body fluids.

Blood

Content in each molecule of hemoglobin: 870 atoms

ROLE

- Vital element; absence causes death
- Provides energy for all life processes

MEDICINAL USES [195]

- Cases of hypoxia, shock, depressive states, poisoning, drowning etc.
- Used for diving operations and high altitude climbing
- Oxygenated water has been used for the treatment of gastric ulcers

TOXICITY [200]

- Life saving O_2 is very toxic in pure form. At 100% atmospheric pressure, it is toxic to alveoli and pulmonary capillaries. Proliferative changes may develop in capillary walls within few hours
- Alveolar hemorrhage
- Trachitis. Reduction in vital capacity of lungs
- Unbearable substernal distress after 48-72 hours
- Depresses natural respiration
- Fire hazard. Flame burns in upper respiratory tract. Bronchoconstriction
- Hyperbaric O_2 therapy may lead to embolus formation and cortical blindness
- Reactive oxygen species (O_2^-, OH; H_2O_2) cause oxidative damage. These have been linked to many pathological conditions

PALLADIUM (Pd)

CATEGORY

Non-essential accumulative ultra-trace element.

DISTRIBUTION IN ECOSYSTEM [118]

Roadside dust	0.2 ppm

HUMAN BODY [93,193]

Presence reported in blood and muscles.

TOXICITY [118]

No information is available on toxic effects of Pd. Possible sources of contamination are from its usage as Pd contacts in electrical engineering.

PHOSPHORUS (P)

CATEGORY

Essential bulk element. Constituent of the basic structure of human body.

HUMAN BODY [15,93,158,200,210,211]

Whole Body Content

- 2.2 million atoms per billion atoms
- 0.8 - 1.2% of body weight
- 1% of total weight of protoplasm
- 12 g/kg of fat-free tissues
- 11,000 ppm
- Total content in average adult man (60 kg): 780 g

Distribution

- Component of all cells and important metabolites: phospholipids, nucleic acids, RNA, DNA, ATP.
- Presence reported in >49 tissues and body fluids.
- 85% of total body P is present in inorganic phase in bones and teeth. Ratio of Ca: P is 2: 1 in bones and teeth, higher P in soft tissues.

ROLE [58,200]

- Provides rigidity to bones and teeth
- Nerve impulse transmission
- Muscle contraction
- Metabolism of carbohydrates, proteins and fats
- Energy supply (ATP), growth and repair processes
- Constituent of enzymes essential for tissue respiration.

DEFICIENCY [58,200]

Causes

Dietary deficiency of P is unlikely. Deficiency may occur from metabolic dysfunction and in patients on prolonged antacid therapy.

Symptoms

- Rickets in children. Osteomalacia in adults
- General weakness
- Decreased phagocytosis
- Depressed cardiac function
- Neurological syndrome
- Respiratory failure

Laboratory Tests

- Serum P analysis
- X ray: osteopenia

INTAKE [41,209]

	P mg/day
Median percentile intake (WHO)	1300
Range of intakes (IAEA)	630-1600
Average intake (China)	1058 ± 397

TOXICITY [77,118,200,209]

- Organophosphate pesticides constitute a major source of P toxicity. These are absorbed by inhalation or skin contact, inhibit choline estrase and interfere in nerve impulse transmission. Some tri-alkyl phosphates (particularly triorthocresyl phosphate), used in plastic industry, in addition cause demyelination. Agricultural workers in developing countries are particularly at risk mainly through sprayinhg pesticides without adequate protection. The risk is aggravated by heat exposure and malnutrition.
- It is a very poisonous element (lethal dose: 1 mg/kg po). Severe symptoms have been reported following ingestion of 15 mg in adults and death with just 3 mg in a two-year child. Symptoms include gastro-intestinal disturbances, hemorrhages, hepatic damage, coma and death. As low dose as 60 mg may be fatal.

- Low serum Ca: P ratio stimulates secondary hyperparathyroidism and result in bone loss. High Ca or PO_4 intake (2g/day) increases fecal output by upto 15% and reduces its bioavailability.
- Fatty foods should be avoided in cases of poisoning.

MEDICINAL USES [77,79,118,140,195]

- Phosphates are incorporated in nervine tonic formulations without much therapeutic justification.
- Phosphates are used for treating osteoporosis. Sodium phosphate has been used to diminish hypercalcaemia.
- Rodenticide
- Smoke screen in war
- ^{35}P has been used in cases of polycythemia vera and granulocytic leukemia.
- Diagnostic uses have been reported in bone disorders, liver disease and metastatic carcinoma of the prostate.

PLATINUM (Pt)

CATEGORY

Non-essential accumulative ultra-trace element.

DISTRIBUTION IN ECOSYSTEMS [118]

Sea water	100-200 × 10^{-6} ppb
Dust (San Diego, California)	0.6-0.8 ppm

HUMAN BODY [15,93,193]

	Pt μg/l
Blood	< 40
Serum	< 100
	Pt μg/gf
Heart	0.0007

ROLE/ESSENTIALITY

Platinum has no physiological role in the body.

DEFICIENCY

As Pt is a non-essential element, there is no known deficiency syndrome/disease.

GUIDELINE VALUES [118]

	Pt mg/m³
Occupational Exposure Limit (German MAK, US Threshold value)	0.002-1.0

MEDICINAL USES [15,118]

(*a*) Cisplatinum compounds are reported to elicit antibacterial, anti-viral and anti-tumour activity both in animals and man. Cisplatinum and carbaplatinum compounds are used for chemotherapy of cancer.

(*b*) Platinum and its alloys have been used in dental amalgams.

TOXICITY [15,81,118]

Sources of Exposure/Contamination

From household, medical and industrial uses in:

(*a*) Jewellary

(*b*) Dentistry

(*c*) Scientific equipment

(*d*) Petroleum refining

(*e*) Industrial catalyst

(*f*) Cancer therapy

Signs/Symptoms

- Allergic dermatitis, urticaria
- Corrhyza-like syndrome, asthma, dyspnoea
- Renal damage
- Myelosuppression

- Irreversible ototoxicity (tinnitus and hearing loss) has been reported following exposure to Cisplatin.
- The element has been shown to cause chromosomal damage in human cell cultures.

MECHANISM OF TOXICITY

Myelosuppression

TREATMENT [15]

(*a*) Control of dust exposure through washing of the affected area reduces the chances of occupational allergy.

(*b*) Symptomatic treatment – Osmotic diuretics with vigourous prehydration
– Adrenaline injections
– Oxygen administration
– Nervine tonics/Vitamins etc.

POLONIUM (Po)

CATEGORY

Non-essential accumulative ultra-trace element.

HUMAN BODY [93,193]

Presence has been reported in whole blood, bones, hair and dentine of teeth.

TOXICITY [118]

It is attributed with mutagenic and carcinogenic properties, Po in cigarette smoke may result in irradiation of lungs and lung cancer.

POTASSIUM (S)

CATEGORY

Essential bulk element.

DISTRIBUTION IN ECOSYSTEMS [118]

	K µg/g Mean (Range)
Soil	2.50 (1.83-3.24)

HUMAN BODY [15,93,158,210,211]

Whole Body Content

- 570,000 atoms per billion atoms.
- 2.6 g/kg body weight
- 0.35% of total weight of protoplasm
- 69 m Eq/kg of fat-free tissues
- 2000 ppm
- Total content in average adult man (60 kg): 140-150 g

Distribution

- Present in almost all tissues and body fluids (reported in > 54)
- Principal cation of the intracellular fluid
- Exchangeable K^+ shows sex differences (more in males vs. females)

ROLE [182,200]

- Regulation of – Cell membrane transfer
  - Osmolarity
  - pH
- Nerve muscle function
- Na^+/K^+ ATP-ase
- Essential in enzyme systems for carbohydrate and protein metabolism.
- Its metabolism is regulated by aldosterone. A small (as small as 0.1 m Eq/l) increase or decrease stimulates or depresses aldosterone production and secretion.

DEFICIENCY [200]

Causes

- Dietary deficiency is unlikely.

- Conditioned deficiency may occur in illness/injury:
  - Renal disease/diuretic therapy
  - Diabetic acidosis
  - Diarrhoea/excessive vomiting
  - Hyperfunction of adrenal cortex
  - Chronic lung disease etc.

Symptoms

- Gastrointestinal disturbances
- Anorexia
- Polyurea
- Apathy, mental confusion, lassitude, depression
- Paralysis
- Edema

Laboratory Tests

- Low serum and urinary K^+
- Abnormal ECG
- Low body K (using ^{40}K)

Other Uses

Level of K has been found to reflect body composition. Exchangeable K is used to compute fat free body weight.

INTAKE REQUIREMENTS [209]

- Median percentile intake (WHO) : 2670 mg/day.
- Range of intakes (IAEA) : 2300 - 3900 mg/day
- Safe and adequate intake levels for K are as follows :

		K mg/day
Infants	upto 6 months	350 - 925
	6 months to 1 year	425 - 1275
Children	1 to 3 years	550 - 1650
	4 to 6 years	775 - 2325

7 to 10 years	1000 - 3000
> 11 years	1525 - 4575
Adults	1875 - 5625

Fruits and vegetables are good sources for K

MEDICINAL USES [77,79,190,195]

Chloride

(*i*) To control cardiac manifestations of digitalis poisoning

(*ii*) Loss associated with diuretic drugs

(*iii*) Periodic familial paralysis

(*iv*) Hypercalcaemia

(*v*) Myasthenia gravis

Citrate

(*vi*) Antacid

Iodide

(*vii*) Antiseptic

Permangnate

(*viii*) Germicidal

Sodium tartrate

(*ix*) Emetic

(*x*) Cathartic

Perchlorate

(*xi*) Thyrotoxicosis

Insulin and Dextrose Infusion

(*xii*) Angina pectoris

TOXICITY [77]

- Small bowel ulcers
- Excess K may be a problem in cases of acidosis and renal failure
- Arrhythmias, cardiac arrest, death

PRASEODYMIUM (Pr)

CATEGORY

Non-essential accumulative ultra-trace element.

DISTRIBUTION ECOSYSTEMS [118]

Earth's crust	8.2 ppm

HUMAN BODY [93,193]

Presence has been detected in tooth enamel.

TOXICITY [118]

Pr nitrate, given i.v., was shown to be highly toxic in rats. Male rats were less susceptible vs. female rats.

PROCTACTINIUM (Pa)

CATEGORY

Not reported in human body

PROMETHIUM (Pm)

CATEGORY

Not reported in human body.

RADIUM (Ra)

CATEGORY

Non-essential accumulative ultra-trace element.

HUMAN BODY [93,193]

Presence reported in whole blood, plasma, bones, heart, liver, kidneys, spleen, testes, skeletal muscles, skin and hair.

GUIDELINE VALUES [118]

Occupational Exposure Limit for ^{226}Ra

Inhalation	:	2×10^4 Bq
Ingestion	:	7×10^4 Bq

MEDICINAL USES [15]

Sealed-in-tubes, needles, plaques and moulds of ^{226}Ra are clinically used for irradiation in carcinomas of buccal mucosa, cheeks, tongue, larynx, anal canal, uterus, vagina, eyes and ears. Beta and gamma rays from Ra are used for surface application in *Cavernous hemangioma* and *Epithelioma.*

TOXICITY [15,118,193]

Radium is readily absorbed from gastrointestinal tract (20%) because of its high solubility. The target organ is the skeleton with a very long biological half-life (20 years). Indoor environment and tobacco smoke may contain Ra. High concentrations have been reported in aquatic systems because of leaching of Ra from any source. This is of great concern. Like all other substances causing ionizing radiation, Ra is mutagenic, carcinogenic and teratogenic. Prolonged retention in bones is particularly alarming. The adverse effects of ^{226}Ra include bone sarcomas, (with a body burden of 50μg Ra), leukemias, developmental defects, impaired brain function and mental retardation. The metal finally decays to noble gas Rn with a short half life (3.8 days) and is eliminated from the body.

RADON (Rn)

CATEGORY

Non-essential accumulative ultra-trace element.

HUMAN BODY [93,193]

Detected in whole blood.

GUIDELINE VALUES [118]

Occupational Exposure Limit for ^{222}Rn on inhalatory exposure: 7×10^6 Bq

TOXICITY [118]

Noble gas Rn (half life: 3.8 days) may escape from subsoil, drinking water and building materials to reach critical levels in the environment. Miners may be exposed to high concentrations. Presence is also reported in indoor environment. Target organ is the lung and exposure to ^{222}Rn may cause lung cancer. Tracheobronchial and pulmonary regions deposits may occur on attachment of ^{222}Rn to ^{214}Pb and ^{214}Po. This causes localized irradiation which is hazardous.

RHENIUM (Re)

CATEGORY

Non-essential accumulative ultra-trace element.

HUMAN BODY [93,193]

Presence reported in whole blood, serum and tooth enamel.

RHODIUM (Rh)

CATEGORY

Non-essential accumulative ultra-trace element.

HUMAN BODY [93,193]

Presence reported in whole blood, serum lungs and dental enamel.

GUIDELINE VALUES [118]

Occupational limit for Rh aerosols	0.1 mg/m^3 air

TOXICITY [118]

While Rh compounds are often used as exhaust catalysts in automobile industry, no reports are available for its toxic effects.

RUBIDIUM (Rb)

CATEGORY

Possibly essential trace element

DISTRIBUTION IN ECOSYSTEM [158]

Earth's crust	100 ppm
Sea water	120 ppb

HUMAN BODY [93,118,158,209]

Whole Body Content

- Total number of atoms : 7.9×10^{21}
- Atoms in each cell : 7.9×10^{7}
- Total content in average adult man (60 kg) : approx. 1.1 g

Blood

Whole blood of children : 12 ± 3 ppm

Distribution

Widely distributed. Presence reported in >38 human tissues and body fluids.

Content : Liver 0.4 – 6 mg/kg, Whole blood 2-4 mg/l, Serum 0.1 – 0.3 µg/l, Urine 1 – 4 mg/day, Milk 0.3 – 1.2 mg/l, Hair 1 – 2 mg/kg.

ROLE [195,200]

Role is not known. Some indicators are given below:

- Metabolism of Rb and Cs is closely related to that of K. Interchangeable with K with little evidence of toxicity.
- Significant increase in serum Rb concentrations has been reported in uremia patients.
- Patients with alcohol abuse revealed 30% less Rb in brain nuclei vs. normal subjects.
- Higher Rb concentrations were reported in cases of breast tumour vs. normal breast tissue.
- ATPase is activated even by low concentrations of Rb
- Brain slices treated with high Rb concentrations show increased oxygen uptake.

INTAKE/REQUIREMENTS [209]

Median percentile intake (WHO)	2.2 mg/day
Requirements	Not known

MEDICINAL USES

Rb chloride is reported to be useful in cases of hypertension.

TOXICITY [118]

e.g., with Daunorubicin

- Stomatitis
- Cardiomyopathy, ECG changes
- Renal damage
- Bone marrow depression. Aplastic anaemia
- Chromosomal damage

RUTHENIUM (Ru)

CATEGORY

Non-essential accumulative ultra-trace element.

HUMAN BODY [93,193]

Presence reported in whole blood, serum, lungs and dental enamel.

TOXICITY [118]

Exposure to Ru may occur from its use in electro-chemical industry. It is considered close to Pb in physiological incompatibility with living cells. Toxic effects may be manifested in kidneys, liver, spleen, mucus membranes and the nervous system. Detailed reports are not available.

SAMARIUM (Sm)

CATEGORY

Non-essential accumulative ultra-trace element.

DISTRIBUTION IN ECOSYSTEMS [118]

	Sm ppm
Earth's crust	6.00
Soil	3.90

HUMAN BODY [93,193]

Presence reported in many tissues and body fluids e.g., whole blood, serum, heart, lungs, diaphragm, lymph nodes, bones, skin, dental enamel etc.

TOXICITY [118]

Administration of Sm nitrate i.v. to female rats was shown to be highly toxic, male rats were less susceptible to Sm toxicity.

SCANDIUM (Sc)

CATEGORY

Non-essential accumulative ultra-trace element.

DISTRIBUTION IN ECOSYSTEMS [118]

Soil	6.84 ppm

HUMAN BODY [93,193]

Presence has been reported in whole blood, serum, brain, heart, liver, bones, skin, tooth enamel, milk and urine.

INTAKE/REQUIREMENTS [209]

Median percentile intake (WHO) : 0.38 mg/day

As it is a non-essential element, there are no known requirements for Sc

No reports available on metabolism and toxicity.

SELENIUM (Se)

CATEGORY

- Possibly essential ultra-trace element.
- Situated immediately below S in the periodic table, occurs wherever S occurs and there is close similarity in chemical reactivity between the two elements.

DISTRIBUTION IN ECOSYSTEM [15,49,118]

Widely distributed in earth's crust, air, water plants and food. Content in food is 100 times less than that in soil. It is present in food in combination with S as selenomethionine, selenocysteine, selenotaurine, selenomethylmethionine, dimethyl-selenures etc.

AIR	**Se mg/m^3**
Permissible level at work place	< 0.2
WATER	**Se mg/Kg**
River water	0.20
Sea water	0.09

Groundwater: Se may get mobilized into it from the soil under acidic conditions. Consumption and use of such water should be restricted to protect public health. A recent survey revealed Se levels in Delhi to be marginally above the specified Indian standards.

SOIL	**Se mg/kg**
Mean (Range)	0.4 (0.1 to 1.0)

PLANT FOODS [118]

	Se mg/kgf
Cereals	0.025-0.38
Potatoes	0.025
Vegetables	0.027
Fruits	0.023
Mushrooms	0.03-13.0
Tea	0.04
Coffee	0.034

ANIMAL FOODS [118]

	Se /kg d
Milk	10-100g
Beef	0.35 mg
Pork	0.52 mg
Chicken	0.21 mg
Eggs	1.8 mg
Organ meats (liver, kidney)	1.57-5.97 mg
Fish	1.4 - 2.9 mg

HUMAN BODY [14,36,93,158,195]

Whole Body Content

- 1.5×10^{20} atoms in the body.
- 1.5×10^{6} atoms in each cell
- 0.2 ppm
- Content in average adult (60 kg): approx. 10-20 mg

Distribution

- Distribution in more than 30 tissues and body fluids including vital organs with relatively higher concentrations in brain, kidneys, testes, ovaries, endocrine glands, hair and nails.

- **Blood**

	Se µg/L
Whole blood	57-320 (171)
RBCs	71-340
Plasma	< 30-590
Serum	98-327 (122)

- **Tissues**

	Se µg/g ash
Brain	0.27-1.64 f
Heart	0.18-1.14 f
Liver	1.73-2.40 d
Kidneys	3.5 d
Lungs	0.23 f
Skin	0.27 f

ROLE/ESSENTIALITY [29,50,59,97,177,200,209]

- ***History:*** Earlier known only for its toxic and carcinogenic effects. The turning point was discovery of its essentiality in rats in 1957. Later it was shown to elicit protective action against skin cancer in mice. The real breakthrough came with the discovery that Se is a constituent of glutathione peroxidase in early seventies.

- ***Constituent of Glutathione peroxidase (GPx) and Factor 3***

  Each molecule of GPx contains 4 organically-bound Se atoms. This enzyme protects against lipid peroxidation and cytotoxicity.

- Selenium has been shown to prevent hepatic necrosis in vitamin-E deficient rats.

- ***Role in biological oxidation/reduction processes***

  The nature of participation in electron transfer, however, is not fully understood.

- ***Intracellular synthesis***

  Living cells regulate Se concentrations by complicated biochemical pathways involving organic Se compounds synthesized intracellularly.

- ***Low content in diseases***

  Though precise cause/effect relationship has not been established, lower Se levels were observed in many diseases *e.g.*, cirrhosis, kwasiorkor, diabetes, cataract, renal ailments, cancer and also in patients under hemodialysis and carbamazepine treatment.

- **Nutritional Role** for Se has been reported in many pathological conditions (heart disease, arthritis, muscular dysfunction, cystic fibrosis, cataract, sexual dysfunction) and aging.

- ***Relationship with Vitamin E:*** Both Se and Vitamin E are micronutrients which have been shown to prevent hepatic necrosis (mice, rats, pigs), exudative diatheses (chicks), muscular dystrophy (animals: species variation), infertility and encephalopathy (human beings). Symptoms of Se deficiency may resemble those of Vitamin-E deficiency partly or wholly.

- ***Detoxicant :*** Se inhibits toxicity of As, Cd, Hg.

- ***Synthesis of tri-idothyronine from thyroxine:*** Involvement of a selenoenzyme has been shown.

DEFICIENCY [50,59,90,118,177,195,200,209]

ANIMALS

Deficiency syndrome has been described both in experimental and farm animals, rat, guinea pig, rabbit, hamster, poultry, dog, sheep, goat, swine, cattle and monkey. The symptoms include retarded growth, infertility, hepatic necrosis, cystic and pancreatic fibrosis, renal degeneration, loss of hair/feathers and gizzard myopathy. **Stiff lamb disease** is attributed to Se deficiency.

HUMAN BEINGS

Negative health effects may occur at Se intake levels below 20 μg/day. Selenium deficient populations (China, Newzealand, Finland etc.) suffered from three specific diseases: **(*i*) Keshan's disease, (*ii*) Kaschin Beck disease, and (*iii*) Neuronal ceroid lipofuscinosis.** In addition its deficiency has been linked to many other human ailments *e.g.*, Ischemic heart disease, Mulberry heart disease, Multiple sclerosis, Hepatocellular carcinoma, Muscular degeneration/pain, Arthritis, Periodontal disease, Diabetic retinopathy, Protein energy malnutrition etc. Laboratory tests for Se deficiency are (*a*) reduced plasma/RBC levels of Se and (*b*) depressed GPx activity particularly in platelets. The latter is the best index for Se status.

KESHAN'S DISEASE

- Cardiomyopathy is endemic in China in a belt stretching between Northeast to Southwest part of the country and gets its name from Keshan district with high incidence.
- It affected a population of about 50 million and thousands died. The population was found to be Se deficient with an average intake of 11 µg/day in contrast to normal intake values in the range of 50 to 200 µg/day elsewhere and RDA of 70 µg/day. Serum Se levels of affected population were less than 10 µg/l. Migrants belt did not suffer.
- Women and children are more susceptible to this disease and more cases were reported in winter season.
- Symptoms included acute or chronic cardiac insufficiency, irregular pulse, ECG changes e.g. gallop arrhythmia.
- Four types: (*i*) Acute (cardiogenic shock), (*ii*) Subacute, (*iii*) Chronic (low output/pump failure), and (*iv*) Latent (No discernible symptoms, minor heart enlargement).
- Post-mortem histopathology: fibrosis of myocardium, multi-focal necrosis.
- Intensive collaborative research by team of Chinese, German and American scientists revealed low blood Se levels.
- Mass-scale supplementation programme with Se enriched salts or sodium selenite tablets (1 mg Se per week) yielded positive results with reduction of incidence to less than one per 100,000 population since 1978.

KASCHIN BECK DISEASE

- Endemic in rural population Se deficient regions of China adjacent to Keshan's district in East Siberia.
- Painful disabling osteoarthropathy with breakdown of collagen-affecting joints. Inflammatory symptoms in initial stages may lead to degenerative osteoarthrosis.
- Children are more prone to the disease.
- Multifactor etiology suspected. Supplementation of Se in combination with Vitamins A and C is more effective in its management. Some reports attribute the disease to a virus.
- Selenium probably is beneficial by functioning as a booster for immune function.

METABOLISM [27,50,59,209]

Absorption

- Absorption occurs both from oral and inhalatory routes.
- Most of the oral absorption takes place from duodenal part of the gastrointestinal tract.

Binding/Metabolism

- It is a component of about 13 selenoproteins and selenopeptides including selenomethionine and selenocysteine as also many enzymes *e.g.*, GPx, glycine reductase, muscle cytochromes etc.
- Bound forms are distributed by circulation to all tissues and body fluids.
- GPx, which constitutes 40% of the total Se, is its functional form.
- Reduction is followed by methylation. Biological half life is 14.4 days.
- Both blood-brain and placental barriers are crossed.

Excretion

- Excretion occurs through feces, urine (methylated derivatives) and expired air. The latter is the main route of excretion at high levels of exposure.
- High content of P, proteins, methionine in diet enhances its renal and pulmonary excretion.

MEDICINAL USES [50,55,79,88,144,195,220]

1. ***Keshan's disease:*** In a four-year study in the Sichun province of China, mass supplementation with Se (0.5-1.0 mg once a week), marked protection was observed against this disease. Both the incidence and mortality rates were significantly reduced.
2. ***Congestive heart failure:*** In a 61-year-old cancer patient on total parenteral nutrition (TPN) for 8 months, addition of selenious acid (40 μg/day) in the TPN solution lead to marked clinical/radiological improvement within a week and digoxin doses could be reduced.
3. ***Cancer Prevention:*** Current evidence and research needs were recently reviewed.[43] A remarkably consistent body of scientific data exists on animal tumour and cell culture models and some epidemiological studies. Clinical trial data is less extensive but it is also supportive.[43,173]
4. ***Miscellaneous:*** Beneficial effects have been reported following Se therapy in various diseases including atherosclerosis, viral hepatitis, arthritis, kwashiorkor, HIV infection, depressed immune function, cancer and by local application in skin diseases. It is reported to reduce the adverse side effects of anticancer drugs Cisplantin and Adriamycin without affecting their anti-cancer activity.

INTAKE/REQUIREMENTS [50,209]

	Se µg/day
Safe and adequate intake (WHO)	
Children 1-3 years	20-80
4-6 years	30-120
>7 years	50-200
Recommended Dietary Allowance (RDA)	70
Maximum safe intake level	400

GUIDELINE VALUES [118,209]

Drinking water	Se mg/L
Permissible limit (WHO)	0.01
Excessive (Min. of Health, Government of India)	0.05
Occupational exposure limit (40 h work week)	0.2 mg/m^3
Biological exposure limit	
Blood	400 mg/g
Urine	5-30 µg/L
Listed by EP under hazardous waste category	

TOXICITY [15,50,118,177]

Sources of Exposure/Contamination

Through industrial and common uses in:

(*a*) Glass and paint industries for neutralizing green colour due to Fe impurities.

(*b*) Plastic and ceramic industries. Sulfoselenide pigment (yellow/maroon).

(*c*) Electronic equipment due to its semiconducting properties.

(*d*) Vulcanizing of rubber

(*e*) Photocopying/xerographic materials

(*f*) Photoelectric cells

(*g*) Pharmaceuticals/cosmetics insecticides/fungicides, antioxidant, anti-dandruff agents.

(*h*) Diagnostic scanning and labeling agent for malignant tumours.

ANIMALS

- **Experimental animals:** Selenotoxicity has been shown in rats, hamsters, rabbits. It is manifested by the following symptoms: anorexia, enteritis, growth depression, weight loss, hepatic and renal damage, postural defects, paralysis of hind quarters, reduced fertility and teratogenic effects.
- **Farm Animals: Blind staggers** is a specific disease due to excess Se in farm animals. It is manifested by dyspnoea, garlic odour from breath, hyperventilation, pulmonary edemas, ascites, emesis, diarrhoea, tachycardia, ataxia, incoordination and death. Another disease in farm animals is **Alkali disease** with symptoms of growth depression, diarrhoea, laboured breathing, prostration, hoof malformation, lameness, low B.P. and hemoglobin level, atrophic damage to liver and heart muscle and ascites.

MAN

- Fortunately man is less sensitive to Se toxicity vs. farm animals.
- Industrial exposure to fumes may show toxic manifestations *e.g.*, metallic taste, lassitude, fatigue, dental decay, gastrointestinal disturbances, irritation to mucus membrane of eyes and respiratory passages, dizziness and pyrexia.
- **Selenotoxicosis** was reported in Enshi region of China with symptoms of brittle hair and nails, prolonged prothrombin time, garlic odour from breath, icteroid skin, dermatitis, inflammation of mucus membranes, headache, heartburn, convulsions and death. High blood/hair content and urinary Se excretion was observed in affected people.
- Skin contact may cause dermatitis, painful penetration under nails, burns, pink eyelids and rosy eyes.
- Toxicity depends on chemical form of Se; selenious acid is most toxic.

SYSTEMIC EFFECTS [118,195,200]

1. *Liver:* Selenium, as a constituent of Factor 3, plays a **protective role against hepatic necrosis.** Low serum Se levels are observed in alcoholism, hepatitis, cirrhosis including Indian childhood cirrhosis, hepatic necrosis, kwashiorkor and Hodgkin's disease. The deterioration of liver function, irrespective of etiology, is accompanied by reduction in serum Se concentrations.
2. *Kidneys:* **Nephrosis** is a manifestation of Se toxicity. Low Se levels have been reported in many renal diseases including **Maple syrup urine disease** in infants (patients: 2.8 μg/L, healthy infants of the same age group: 18-112 μg/L).

3. ***Nervous system:*** Symptoms of Se intoxication include polyneuritis manifested by 'pins and needles' sensation, paraesthesia, numbness, pain in extremities, motor disturbances, paralysis, convulsions and death. **Neuronal ceroid lipofuschinosis (NCL)**, a neurodegenerative disease, is attributed to Se deficiency.

4. ***Cardiovascular system:*** Symptoms of chronic selenosis include anaemia, palpitation and complaints of heart burn. Autopsy samples of patients dying of cardiovascular diseases show significantly low Se concentrations. Marked decline in selenoenzyme GPx has been reported in cases of thrombasthenia. Deficiency states result in increased sensitivity to oxidative damage to membranes and oxidant sensitive proteins *e.g.*, hemoglobin. Lowest death rates from cardiovascular diseases were associated with highest Se levels in heart muscle samples from Philippines and vice versa from USA. Blood platelets, with highest Se concentrations (782 ±127 mg/g fresh weight) are considered crucial for triggering thrombosis and so such analyses are important for clinical cardiology.

5. ***Respiratory system:*** Inhalatory exposure causes irritation/inflammation of mucus membranes of respiratory passages and garlic odour from breath.

6. ***Skin:*** Medicinal uses (selenium sulphide 2.5%) have been reported in skin diseases (seborrhoeic dermatitis, psorariform seborrhoea, acne vulgaris, eczema) and in antidandruff shampoos. Thorough washing of hands/nails should be done after each application to prevent dermal absorption and systemic toxicity.

7. ***Reproductive system:*** It is needed for normal reproductive function. Regulatory processes ensure preferential supply in testes, high concentration in sperms, conservation (decreased urinary excretion) during pregnancy and accumulation in fetal liver.

8. ***Immune function:*** Selenium potentiates immune response. This is evidenced by: (*a*) increased T-cell-dependent antibody response and (*b*) enhanced natural killer cell activity. Patients of AIDS have been reported to be Se deficient. Protective action against spontaneous and transplantable tumour induction was observed following nutritional supplementation with this element.

MECHANISM OF TOXICITY [15,118]

- Ability to block the protective action of SH group of enzymes and S containing amino acids.
- Strong interactions with nutrients Vitamin C and E.

TREATMENT [15,118]

- Elimination of source of contamination/exposure.
- Local application of 10% sodium thiosulphate on burns caused by Se dioxide and use of desensitizing drugs.
- Use of chelating agents dimercaprol and disodium calcium EDTA should be avoided as these may enhance Se toxicity.
- No specific antidotes are available for the treatment of patients exposed to compounds containing selenious acid (*e.g.*, gum-bluing solution)
- Symptomatic treatment and supportive measures *e.g.*, intravenous fluids, oxygen etc. are helpful.

SILICON (Si)

CATEGORY

- Possibly essential bulk element.

FOOD [209]

Plant origin food items contain more Si vs. animal origin food.

HUMAN BODY [33,93,158,195,200]

Whole Body Content

- 260 ppm
- Total content in average adult man (60 kg): 18 g
- Content decreases with age

Distribution

- Widely distributed
- Reference values for serum Si were recently established at the Department of Clinical Chemistry, University Hospital, Freiburg, Germany. The study involved determination of serum Si concentrations in 1325 healthy adults (18-91 yrs) using atomic absorption spectrometry.[33] The median values showed age and sex dependency as follows:

Sex	Age (Years)	Median Serum Si concentration (μ mol/L)
Men	18-59	9.50
	60-74	8.50
	> 74	7.70
Women	18-29	10.00
	30-44	11.10
	45-59	9.23
	> 74	8.00

- Presence reported in > 30 human tissues and body fluids
- Mucopolysaccharides and fibres in connective tissue contain higher Si concentrations (> 100 μg/g) vs. other organs/tissues *e.g.*, liver, lungs, muscles, brain (2-10 μg/g)

ROLE [108,120,187,200,209]

- Major ion of osteogenic cells specially in metabolically active stage.
- Role in bone calcification and cross linking of connective tissue particularly in bone cartilage.
- **Atherosclerosis:** Si content in aorta decreases with aging and development of atherosclerosis. Large i.v. doses in cholesterol fed rabbits were shown to reduce incidence of this disease.
- A recent report,[68] on elderly osteoporotic women (≥ = 75 yrs) from five geographic areas of France, revealed that low Si concentrations were associated with low cognitive performance at baseline. Silicon in drinking water may reduce the risk of developing **Alzheimer's disease**. The potential therapeutic value of silica for cognitive impairment needs to be confirmed by further studies.

DEFICIENCY [118,120,187,200,209]

- **Experimental animals:** Deficiency states in chicken and rat showed the following symptoms:
  - (*i*) Growth retardation

(*ii*) Weak bones with reduction in matrix component. Bone deformities in skull and peripheral bones

(*iii*) Structural changes in cells

(*iv*) Poor pigmentation

(*v*) Seborrhoea

(*vi*) Atony

The symptoms could be reversed by Si supplementation.

- ***Man:*** Human deficiency has not been reported. The possibility exists with increasing use of refined foods. The content is more in plant foods vs. animal origin food items. Grains and citrus fruits are particularly rich sources.

INTAKE/REQUIREMENTS [209]

- *Estimated daily intake for adults:* 10-50 mg
- *Requirement:* Experimental Animals 100-250 μg/g of diet

  Human beings: Precise requirements are not available.

MEDICINAL USES [50,52,109,200,209]

- Potential for therapeutic utility in atherosclerosis needs further investigations.
- Protective effect of Si was demonstrated in cases of simple myopia in children.
- Amorphons Si flat panel imaging devices for dosimetry purposes.

TOXICITY/SILICOSIS [21,200,209]

- Relatively less toxic. Dust inhalation may lead to **pneumoconiosis.**
- Inhalation or ingestion of large amounts over prolonged period (10-15 years) has been reported to develop **fiberous nodules in lungs.** In advanced stages, 50% cases may become infected with tuberculosis.
- Kidney damage, nephropathy and urolithiasis.
- Asbestos (a silicate mineral) is known to be carcinogenic
- A comparative study on 332 industrial workers in Iran (pottery, ceramic, stone other and stone grinder factories) revealed adverse effects of Si dust on lung function.[21] Forced expiratory volume in one second (FEV 1) and Forced vital capacity (FVC) were significantly lower among stone-grinders compared with pottery, ceramic in stone cutter workers and the healthy control subjects. The prevalence of respiratory symptoms was higher in stone grinders vs. that in other workers. The concentration of Si particles was 40-100 times higher in these workers. More attention is, therefore, needed to ventilation systems and health care of stone grinders.

SILVER (Ag)

CATEGORY

Non-essential accumulative ultra-trace element.

DISTRIBUTION IN ECOSYSTEMS [15,35,118]

AIR

North America and Europe	1 mg/m^3

WATER

	Ag µg/kg
Sea water	0.0002
River water	0.20

Groundwater: Ag may get mobilized into it from the soil under acidic conditions. Consumption and use of such water should be restricted to protect public health.

SOIL

Surface soil	50 µg/kg

PLANTS [118]

Range of content in land plants	0.06-0.28 µg/g (dry weight)
Aquatic plants accumulate several hundred fold of these values by concentrating Ag from their environment.	
Wheat Bran	0.3 µg/g

ANIMALS/ANIMAL ORIGIN FOODS [15,118]

Mammals	0.006 µg/g f
Beef, Pork, Mutton	11 mg/kg
Liver	0.03 ppm
Brain	0.04 ppm
Kidneys	0.005 ppm
Milk	25-54 mg/l

HUMAN BODY[93]

WHOLE BODY CONTENT

Total content in average adult man (60 kg) 0.1-1 mg

TISSUES/BODY FLUIDS

- Reported in > 40 human tissues and body fluids

	μg/g ash
■ Blood	
Whole blood	3.4 – 120
Serum	2.9 – 200
Erythrocytes	4.3 – 15
■ Tissues	
Bones	1.1
Brain	< 0.5 – 1.7
Liver	< 0.1 – 1.7
Kidneys	< 0.1 – 0.5
Hair	0.025-3.8
	μg/l
■ Urine	10

ROLE/DEFICIENCY [59]

There is no known physiological function or deficiency syndrome for Ag. It competes effectively with Cu and Se in many biological reactions *e.g.*, Ag displaces Cu and interferes with biosynthesis of ceruloplasmin involved in Fe mobilization.

METABOLISM [15,118]

Absorption

Silver can be absorbed through skin, lungs and the gastrointestinal tract. The absorption is poor (oral : 10%, very little pulmonary absorption following accidental inhalation). Substantial absorption may occur from topical application of Ag sulfadiazine during burn therapy. Intact keratin is an effective barrier.

Distribution

Only 10% of absorbed Ag is retained. It is widely distributed and gets fixed in tissues. Retention is greatest in the reticulo-endothelial system. About 9 mg of Ag may be accumulated in 50 years from its normal intake in food and water. Half life in skin is longer vs. other tissues: about 50 days.

Metabolism[13,167]

Silver ion has a great affinity for sulphydryl, amino and phosphate groups. It forms complexes with amino acids, purines, pyramidines, nucleosides, nucleotides, DNA and RNA. Metallothioneins have great affinity for Ag. These biochemical reactions may influence toxicity/detoxification mechanisms.

Excretion

Most of Ag is excreted (90%) primarily in feces and traces in urine.

INTAKE/REQUIREMENTS [17,118]

Total intake from food and water	20-80 μg/day

As it is a non-essential element, there are no known requirements for Ag.

GUIDELINE VALUES [118]

Drinking water standards	**Ag μg/l**
USA	50
Switzerland	200
Safe, stable and long lasting purification of drinking water in Russia	0.1-0.2 ppm Ag ion
	Ag μg/m³
Occupational exposure level in air	0.1

Listed by EP under hazardous waste category

MEDICINAL USES [17-20,152,200]

- ***Burns/Wounds:*** Silver sulfadiazine cream (a topical antibacterial preparation) is used for treating burn victims. Its site of action is the bacterial cell membrane and it is more potent vs. sulfadiazine alone. Silver nitrate (0.5%) dressings (changed 12 hourly) constitute an effective treatment for burns, wounds and sepsis. Other preparations, used for the same purpose, include Ag sulfadiazine dry foam and $AgNO_3$ sprays.
- ***Warts:*** Cautery by $AgNO_3$ is used to remove warts, moles etc.
- ***Dental Amalgams:*** These are widely used as dental fillings and are considered quite safe. Some reports indicate marginal leakage of Ag from these amalgams.
- ***Ayurvedic/Unani Silver Preparations:*** Silver is not used internally in modern medicine. Calcined Ag preparations, prepared by specialized Ayurvedic/Unani techniques, are attributed with diverse therapeutic properties *e.g.*, tonic/rejuvenating (general, nervine, cardiac and sexual tonic) properties and utility in physical and mental weakness, bronchitis, asthma, tuberculosis, sexual debility and neuropsychiatric disorders. These claims have not been investigated. Some recent studies, however, revealed growth-promoting, analgesic, anti-cataleptic, anxiolytic and antiaggressive effects of Ayurvedic *Raupya Bhasma* and

Unani *Kushta Nuqra* in rats and mice. These actions were observed without discernible gross or subtle toxic effects. While this is very interesting, some pro-convulsive effects were also observed with these preparations in experimental models of epilepsy. Their use may be dangerous in epilepsy-prone patients.

TOXICITY [15,17,118]

Sources of Exposure/Contamination

From general, industrial and medical uses:

(*a*) Photographic materials

(*b*) Coinage

(*c*) Jewellery

(*d*) Cutlery

(*e*) Mirrors

(*f*) Electroplating Works

(g) Disinfectants

(*h*) Dental Amalgams etc.

Major Ag-producing countries are Mexico, Peru, Russia, Canada, Australia and USA. Free Ag in nature occurs in a very limited quantity and is not considered a major environmental/health hazard. Argyria (Ag poisoning) has been reported following the use of antismoking lozenges containing Ag acetate and Ag iodide nasal drops. Colloidal Ag is a systemic poison (fatal dose : 50 mg i.v.). Orally 10 g of $AgNO_3$ may be fatal.

SYSTEMIC EFFECTS [17,77,118,195,200]

(*a*) ***Liver:*** Spectrographic analysis revealed a ten-fold increase in hepatic Ag with Cu in Wilson's disease.

(*b*) ***Cardiovascular system:*** Addition of Ag at 900 ppm (as nitrate or acetate) in diet is reported to depress growth, packed cell volume and cause cardiac enlargement in Turkey poults and chicks. Interactions with Cu, Se and Zn may indirectly influence cardiac function. Exposure to Ag nitrate is reported to cause methemoglobinemia.

(*c*) ***Respiratory system:*** Chronic Ag poisoning (Argyria) manifests itself as blue pigmentation of respiratory passages. Cases of acute intoxication, though rare, have been reported with severe injury to the respiratory centers.

(*d*) ***Nervous system:*** Parcelsus recommended the use of Ag compounds for the treatment of diseases of the nervous system because of the belief that insane individuals/lunatics are under the influence of moon godess. The therapeutic use of Ag in epilepsy and lunacy continued till nineteenth century. It has been now abandoned.

(*e*) ***Skin:*** Some Ag compounds (nitrate, allantoinate, sulfadiazine etc.) are used for local antiseptic and caustic effects. Slate blue pigmentation of elastic fibres of skin is a characteristic feature of chronic Ag poisoning. It starts on the face, hands and finger nails which may later spread all over the body. The pigmentation is usually permanent.

(*f*) ***Infections:*** Silver interferes with metabolic functions of the bacterial cells and elicits germicidal effects. Distilled water becomes markedly bactericidal after contact with metallic Ag though the concentration reaches only 1 in 20 million parts. Silver nitrate (1 in 100 concentration) is bactericidal, higher dilutions are bacteristatic. This property of Ag is used for purifying water and topical use in antiseptic dressings for burns and wounds.

(*g*) ***Carcinogenicity:*** Colloidal Ag is carcinogenic. Sub-cutaneous implantation of Ag foil/particles has been shown to induce sarcomas in rodents. The metal does not seem to be a major risk in human beings through contact or ordinary use.

MECHANISM OF TOXICITY [15]

(*a*) Local irritation/corrosive action

(*b*) Antagonism to essential nutrients *e.g.*, Se, Cu (reduced ceruloplasmin synthesis), Vitamins B_{12} and E.

(*c*) Enhancement of lipid peroxidation.

TREATMENT [15]

There is no specific antidote for Ag poisoning. Symptomatic and supportive treatment is given.

SODIUM (Na)

CATEGORY

- Essential bulk element

DISTRIBUTION IN ECOSYSTEM [118]

	Na µg/g Mean (Range)
Soil	1.86 (1.71-2.04)

HUMAN BODY [14,93,158,210,211]

Whole Body Content

- 410,000 atoms per billion atoms
- 1.8g/kg of body weight
- 0.15% of total weight of protoplasm
- 80 m Eq/kg of fat-free tissues
- 1400 ppm
- Total content in average adult man (60 kg): approx. 100g

Distribution

- Present in almost all tissues and body fluids (reported in > 54).
- Major cation of the extracellular fluid, only a small proportion is present inside the cells.

ROLE [118,200]

- Regulation of
  - (*i*) Osmotic equilibrium
  - (*ii*) pH
  - (*iii*) Plasma volume
- Tissue formation
- Nerve impulse transmission
- Muscle contraction
- While K has main role in aldosterone production and metabolism, Na also plays a part.

DEFICIENCY [79,195,200]

Causes

- Na is widely distributed in foods. Chances of a dietary deficiency are very remote.
- Homeostatic control regulates flexible excretion according to needs of the body.
- Conditioned deficiency may occur in dehydrating illness/injury or fluid loss:
  - (*i*) Diarrhoea, dysentery, excessive vomiting, dehydration.
  - (*ii*) Profuse sweating
  - (*iii*) Adrenal insufficiency
  - (*iv*) Renal disease
  - (*v*) Hemorrhage etc.

Symptoms

- Water loss. Low blood volume and BP. Hypovolemic shock.
- Anorexia, apathy, confusion, weakness, muscular cramps
- Oligouria

Laboratory Tests

- Low-serum Na
- High blood N and urea levels

INTAKE/REQUIREMENTS [209]

- Median percentile intake (WHO) : 3.5 g/day. Range (IAEA) : 3.5 - 6.9 g/day
- Safe and adequate intake levels for Na are as follows:

	Na mg/day
Infants	
upto 6 months	115-350
6 months to 1 year	250-750
Children	
1 to 3 years	325-975
4 to 6 years	450-1350
7 to 10 years	600-1800
>11 years	700-2700
Adults	1100-5300 (mean : 4400)

MEDICINAL USES [209]

- Oral rehydration fluid in cases of diarrhoea, dysentery, dehydration.
- Parenteral nutrition : NaCl, dextrose saline etc. for fluid replacement.
- Miscellaneous uses:

– Bicarbonate/Lactate	:	Antacid
– Alginate	:	Demulcent
– Fluoride	:	Dental caries
– Nitrite	:	Angina, cyanide poisoning
– Citrate/Tartrate	:	Anticoagulant
– Salicylate	:	Analgesic etc.

TOXICITY

- More blood volume. Hypertension
- Edema
- Heart failure

STRONTIUM (Sr)

CATEGORY

- Possibly essential trace element/Biostimulant

HUMAN BODY [93,158,176]

Whole Body Content

- Total number of atoms : 1.0×10^{21}
- Atoms in each cell : 1.0×10^{7}
- 4.6 ppm
- Total content in average adult man (60 kg): approx. 140-340 mg

Distribution

- Presence reported in >45 tissues and body fluids.
- 90% of the body burden is in bones. High concentrations have been reported in pigmented parts of the eye.
- Values for content in bones, lungs, aorta increase with age.

ROLE [140,195]

- It belongs to group II A of the Periodic Table with important elements : Ca, Mg.
- In spite of its widespread distribution, no specific role has been attributed to Sr so far. The element received very little attention earlier because of lack of

  (*a*) Motivation and

  (*b*) Means

  Advent of atomic energy brought both these factors (*a*) **Motivation:** Environmental contamination from radio-nucleotides of Sr and (*b*) **Means:** Availability of Atomic Absorption Spectroscopy (AAS) and Isotopes as investigative tools.
- Sr can replace 25% of Ca in chick ration without adverse effects.
- Biostimulatory action. Supplementation at pharmacological levels increases bone density.
- Alterations in disease states:

  – High serum levels in Uremia

  – Low serum levels in Rheumatoid Arthritis.

DEFICIENCY [195]

Experimental Animals

Rats and Guinea pigs.

- Impairment of bone calcification
- Growth depression
- Higher incidence of dental caries.

Man

Human deficiency has not been reported.

INTAKE [209]

Median percentile intake (WHO): 1.5 mg/day

METABOLISM

- Even with small intake, ^{90}Sr is retained in the body. It accumulates in bones.
- Excretion of Sr is preferential to that of Ca. Principal route of excretion is urine.

MEDICINAL USES [15,200]

- Radioactive ^{90}Sr has been used in cases of:

  (*i*) Bone sarcoma

  (*ii*) Eyelid melanoma

  (*iii*) Mycosis fungoides

  Only palliative effect
- Sr bromide in leprosy
- Limited use as an adjuvant to Ca for remineralisation of bones in cases of osteoporosis and tooth decay.

TOXICITY [15]

^{90}Sr is harmful. It gets fixed in bones and is not eliminated easily. Liberal intake of Ca is helpful. The absorption of Ca is 7 times higher vs. Sr, it competes for the same sites. It reduces the risk of Sr absorption.

SULPHUR (S)

CATEGORY

- Essential bulk element.

HUMAN BODY [14,158]

Whole Body Content

- 490,000 atoms per billion atoms
- 0.25% of the total weight of protoplasm
- 2000 ppm
- Total content in average adult man (60 kg): approx. 140g

Blood

Each molecule of hemoglobin contains 8 atoms of S.

Distribution

- Present in cytoplasm of almost all cells
- Keratin is abundant in S content. Hair, skin and nails are rich in S.
- Most of the body S is present in the form of amino acids: cystine, cysteine and methionine.
- It is a constituent of insulin, bile (taurine) and some vitamins (thiamine, biotin).

ROLE [58]

- Synthesis of essential metabolites through S-containing amino acids.
- Oxidation/reduction reactions.
- Blood clotting
- Development of bones, growth and muscle metabolism.
- Detoxification mechanisms.
- Though present in insulin, no links reported with diabetes mellitus
- Interactions occur with several elements *e.g.*, Cd, Cu, Mo, Se etc.

INTAKE/REQUIREMENTS [118]

- Intake is related to protein intake (through S-containing amino acids)
- RDA: 850 mg/day

MEDICINAL USES [195,200]

- Used externally for antiseptic, fungicidal and parasiticidal effects in the form of ointments, lotions and dusting powders for the treatment of acne, boils, scabies, itching, dermatitis, eczema and leprosy. Also used in cases of leucoderma.
- Germicidal fumigant
- Chemical weapon of war
- S mustard has been reported to inhibit experimental tumours.

TOXICITY [77,195]

- Excess cystine predisposes to fatty liver
- Sulphemoglobinemia
- Endogenous cyanosis
- Acid rain is a major environmental problem.

TANTALUM (Ta)

CATEGORY

Non-essential accumulative ultra-trace element.

DISTRIBUTION IN ECOSYSTEMS [118]

Earth's crust	1 ppm
Sea water	< 0.004 ppm

HUMAN BODY [93,193]

Presence reported in whole blood, serum, lymph nodes, gastro-intestinal tract, and tooth enamel.

METABOLISM [118]

Absorption of ingested Ta is very poor. A large portion gets entrapped in walls of the gastrointestinal tract and digestive glands. It has a long biological half life (1-2 years). Excretion occurs mostly in feces within 7 days. Pulmonary clearance of inhaled Ta depends on particle size. Particles of diameter 1 μm have a half life of about 2.1 years and for size 5-10 μm it is 333 days.

GUIDELINE VALUES [118]

Occupational Exposure Limit	5 mg/m³ air

MEDICINAL USES [118]

It is used in clinical medicine for (*a*) diagnostic radiography with better visibility vs. Ba or I, (*b*) medium for bronchography, (*c*) for detection of occult cancer, (*d*) determination of clearance time in patients with chronic obstructive pulmonary disease, (*e*) blood-pool imaging, (*f*) ophthalmic surgery, (*g*) as radio-opaque biomarker and (*h*) in various types of surgical implants.

TOXICITY [118]

Sources of Exposure/Contamination

From its use in:

- Electronic industry
- Diagnostic and surgical applications

ANIMALS

LD_{50} values of some Ta compounds in rats are as follows:

Oxide	8 g/kg p.o.
Chloride	1.9 g/kg p.o.
	75 mg/kg i.p.
Potassium Tantalum Fluoride	2.5 g/kg p.o.
	375 mg/kg i.p.

MAN

Limited toxicity data is available. Mucopurulent discharge and conjunctivitis following orbital implants, urticaria and anaphylactic sensitization reactions. The latter necessitated removal of implant in some cases.

TECHNETIUM (Tc)

CATEGORY

Not reported in human body.

TELLURIUM (Te)

CATEGORY

Non-essential accumulative ultra-trace element.

DISTRIBUTION IN ECOSYSTEMS [118]

Earth's crust	0.01 ppm
Sea water	0.5-125 ppm

HUMAN BODY [93,193]

The element is widely distributed, presence reported in more than 25 human tissues and body fluids including blood and all vital organs. It is concentrated in skeleton.

ROLE/ESSENTIALITY

There is no known nutritional/physiological role or deficiency syndrome for Te

METABOLISM [118]

Absorption

Gastro-intestinal absorption is approximately 10-30%. Inhalatory absorption is more efficient. Absorption also occurs from intact skin.

Binding/Metabolism

It is readily soluble in body fluids and gets distributed to many tissues/organs. Experimental studies in rats revealed 90% retention in erythrocytes. Deposition occurs in lungs, kidneys, central nervous system and bones. Biological half-life is about 3 weeks. It crosses both blood-brain and placental barriers.

Excretion

Excretion occurs in bile, feces, urine and through pulmonary route.

MEDICINAL USES [81]

Therapeutic use in *Seborrhoea capitis.*

INTAKE/REQUIREMENTS [118]

Estimated intake	600 µg/day
	No known requirements.

GUIDELINE VALUES [118]

	Te µg/m³ air
Occupational Exposure Limit	
UK, USA	100
USSR	10
Urine	Less than 1 µg/L

TOXICITY [118]

Sources of Exposure/Contamination

From personal and industrial uses in:

- Thermoelectric and electronic works
- Metallurgic additive to improve characteristics of alloys
- Catalytic processes
- Vulcanization of rubber
- Solar cells
- Chargeable and non-chargeable fuel cells
- Semiconductor raw material
- Medical applications

  Infra-red emitting glasses

  Myocardial scanning

  Potent anti-stickling agent for erythrocytes etc.

ANIMALS

Restlessness, reduced reflexes, convulsions, paralysis, coma, and death. Liver, kidney and CNS show more adverse effects. Impairment of glycogen function and detoxifying mechanisms has been reported in rats following inhalatory exposure. Other effects included normochronic hemolytic anemia, peripheral neuropathy with weakness in hind quarters, ceroid lipofuscinosis, myelinopathy and gonadal toxicity.

MAN

Garlic odour from breath and sweat, metallic taste, intra-dermal deposits, skin lesions, suppression of sweating, bluish-black pigmentation in face and neck region, fatigue and urinary levels >100 µg/L. Cyanosis, vomiting, loss of consciousness and death may occur. Congesion of lungs, liver, spleen, kidneys, fatty infilteration of liver, black deposits in bladder and ureter have been observed on post mortem.

TERBIUM (Tb)

CATEGORY

Non-essential accumulative ultra-trace element.

DISTRIBUTION IN ECOSYSTEMS [118]

Earth's crust	0.9 ppm

HUMAN BODY [93,193]

Presence reported in whole blood, serum, lymph nodes and tooth enamel.

TOXICITY [118]

Mice fed Tb oxide for 3 generations showed no evidence of toxicity. No differences were observed in mortality, morbidity, morphological development, growth rate and reproduction capacity between the treated and control groups.

THALLIUM (Tl)

CATEGORY

Non-essential accumulative trace element.

DISTRIBUTION IN ECOSYSTEMS [118]

Earth's crust	0.1-0.5 ppm
Sea water	0.01-0.016 µg/L
Ambient air	<1 ng/m^3
River water	0.01-1.0 µg/L
Ground water	upto 800 µg/L

PLANT FOODS [15,118]

	Tl mg/kg f
Cereals	0.02-0.08
Potatoes	0.025
Vegetables	0.0005-0.13
Fruits	0.05-0.14
Mushrooms	0.048

ANIMAL FOODS [15,118]

Pork	0.028-0.138
Kidney	0.063-0.244
Eggs	< 0.1-0.7

HUMAN BODY [93,193]

Thallium is widely distributed in 30 human tissues and body fluids including blood, bones, all vital organs, endocrine glands, skin and hair. Kidney and muscles are depot compartments. Hair is a good indicator for biomonitoring of Tl.

METABOLISM [15,118]

Absorption

- Absorption through oral route or inhalation is rapid and substantial (upto 80 100%)
- May also be absorbed on contact with intact skin.

Distribution

Retention in plasma is longer vs. other metals *e.g.*, Ba, Ni or Zn suggesting its cumulative nature. It gets distributed to many tissues, tracer studies using ^{204}Tl indicated tropism of the isotope in the following order:

Kidneys, Testes > Liver > Spleen > Prostate > Brain > Skin, Hair

Metabolism

Competitively replaced by K^+. Binding in the gastro-intestinal tract, helps in its detoxification.

Excretion

Bulk of Tl is excreted (70-90%) in urine and faeces. Excretion in scalp hair helps in forensic diagnosis and control of therapy.

INTAKE/REQUIREMENTS [118]

Intake : Approx. 2 μg/day but in working areas with inhalatory exposure and skin contact, higher values (10.5-12.6 μg/day) have been reported.

Requirements : It is a non-essential element with no minimum nutritional requirements.

GUIDELINE VALUES [118]

Occupational Exposure Limit	0.1 mg/m^3 air
Agricultural soil	5 mg/kg day

MEDICINAL USES [15]

It is used as a pesticide, rodenticide and depilatory agent.

TOXICITY [15,77,118,200]

Sources of Exposure/Contamination

From industrial/medical uses in:

(*a*) Rodenticides

(*b*) Homeopathic medicines

(*c*) Rectifiers

(*d*) Deep-temperature thermometers

(*e*) Scintillation counters

(*f*) Superconductors

(*g*) Electric contacts

(*h*) Safety fuses

(*i*) Optical lenses

(*j*) Photoelectric cells

(*k*) Costume jewellery

(*l*) Anti-detonators

(*m*) Depilatory preparations

(*n*) Medical diagnostics etc.

Toxic Dose

Thallium is a cumulative poison. Average lethal dose is approx. 0.8 to 1.0 g but toxicity varies with the type of compound. Water-soluble compounds (sulphate, acetate, carbonate) are more toxic vs. less water soluble forms (sulphide, iodide). Death is reported with ingestion of just 3.29 mg of Tl sulphate.

Symptoms

Symptoms appear within 12-24 hours of exposure. These include dry mouth, nausea, vomiting, bloody diarrhoea, colic, soreness of gums, rhinorrhoea, dehydration and shock. It produces alopecia and histological changes in skin. Neurological symptoms appear later (after 2-5 days of exposure) *e.g.*, headache, weakness of muscles, lethargy, paraesthesias, delirium, sleeplessness, vision defects, behavioural disorders, choreform movements, convulsions and coma.

MECHANISM OF TOXICITY [77,118]

- Effect on mitochondrial enzyme systems resulting in cell death
- Inhibition of K

DIAGNOSTIC FEATURES [77,118]

- History of exposure.
- Severe gastroenteritis, loss of scalp in axillae, pubic hair and eyebrows.
- A 24-hour urine assay for Tl is a reliable test (Normal concentration : less than 1.5 μg/l, concentrations more than 100 μg/l are considered toxic).
- Analysis of Tl in scalp hair is useful for forensic diagnosis. Dark pigment deposit in hair roots.

TREATMENT [77,118]

(*a*) Remove poison by inducing emesis (within minutes of Tl ingestion), administer charcoal, gastric lavage, cathartics etc.

(*b*) Symptomatic treatment: anticonvulsants for seizure control, i.v. fluids, hemodialysis, hemoperfusion, infusion of potassium iodide or K ferricyanide to displace Tl and supplement K.

(*c*) Administer prussian blue (potassium ferric ferrocyanide) via naso-jejunal tube and continue therapy till urinary Tl excretion is less than 10 μg/24 hours.

(*d*) There is no specific antidote, dimercaprol and other chelating agents have been used with varying success.

THORIUM (Th)

CATEGORY

Non-essential accumulative ultra-trace element.

DISTRIBUTION IN ECOSYSTEMS [118]

	Th ppm
Earth's crust	13.00
Soil	8.15

HUMAN BODY [15,93,193]

Presence reported in whole blood, erythrocytes, serum, lungs, lymph nodes and bones. Injected Th stays life long in body tissues.

ROLE/ESSENTIALITY/DEFICIENCY

There is no known physiological role, essential function or deficiency syndrome for Th.

GUIDELINE VALUES [15,118]

Radiation Exposure Limit for ^{232}Th

Ingestion	3×10^4
Inhalation	1×10^2

MEDICINAL USES [81]

Therapeutic use in *Superficial capillary naevus*

TOXICITY [15,118]

Sources of Exposure/Contamination

From general/industrial uses in:

(*a*) Incandescent mantles

(*b*) Gas lights

(*c*) Alloys to coat tungsten wires and camera lenses

(*d*) Contrast media in X-ray photography

Signs and Symptoms

It is suspected to be carcinogenic causing bone sarcomas and leukemias. Its use as a contrast media in X-ray photography is considered an occupational hazard. The metal, emitting ionizing radiations at high doses, has been shown to be teratogenic; developmental defects and impaired brain-function have been observed both in experimental animals and man.

MECHANISM OF TOXICITY

Ionizing radiation

THULIUM (Tm)

CATEGORY

Non-essential accumulative ultra-trace element.

DISTRIBUTION IN ECOSYSTEMS [118]

Earth's crust	0.5 ppm

HUMAN BODY [93,193]

Presence reported is whole blood, serum, and tooth enamel.

TOXICITY [118]

It interacts with actin and prevents tubule formation. No other information is available.

TIN (Sn)

CATEGORY

- Possibly essential ultra-trace element

HUMAN BODY [38,93,118,158]

Whole Body Content

- Total number of atoms 1.5×10^{20}
- Atoms in each cell 1.5×10^{6}
- 0.2 ppm
- Content in average adult man (60 kg): approx. 30 mg

Distribution

Presence reported in >43 human tissues and body fluids. Preferential bioaccumulation in thymus gland (6 times higher vs. other organs)

ROLE [38,200,209]

- Precise role is yet to be established.
- Constituent of gastrin, lack of this leads to impaired digestion and growth.
- Probably required for tertiary structure of proteins and other components of biological importance.
- Participates in oxidation/reduction processes.
- Role in immune function speculated and needs to be probed.
- Substantial increase (400-600%) was obsreved in blood Sn levels after tumour (*e.g.*, breast cancer) transplantation. The concentration in cancerous tissue was, however, found to be much lower (Healthy breast : 2.36 μg/g, Breast tumour : 0.72 μg/g).

DEFICIENCY [38,200,209]

Experimental Animals

Rats show growth retardation which is corrected by Sn supplementation.

Man

Human deficiency has not been reported.

METABOLISM [15,118,209]

Absorption

(*a*) **Oral:** absorption is very poor (< 5%). It is influenced by oxidation state. Sn (II) is better absorbed vs. Sn (IV). Compounds with short alkyl chains are better absorbed from the gastrointestinal tract.

(*b*) **Skin:** Trialkyl compounds are well absorbed.

(*c*) **Inhalatory:** The extent of absorption through this route has not been worked out.

Metabolism

- **Retention** is generally low. It is more in bones vs. soft tissues. Deposition occurs in lung, liver and kidney.
- **Dealkylation and dearylation** takes place in liver. The metal crosses both blood-brain and placental barriers.
- **Interactions:** Sn interferes with (*a*) Porphyrin and heme biosynthesis, (*b*) Mitochondrial oxidative phosphorylation, (*c*) Activity of δ-amino levulinic acid dehydratase (δ–ALAD), (*d*) Activity of riboflavin, (*e*) Metabolism of Ca, Cu, Fe, Se and Zn.

Excretion

Excretion of Sn is slow; more than 90% of unabsorbed metal is excreted in feces. The absorbed component is excreted via urine, bile, pancreatic juice, milk and sweat.

MEDICINAL USES [195,198]

- Use in tape worm infestation
- Sn coating of brass/copper utensils has been reported to prevent Indian childhood cirrhosis.

INTAKE/REQUIREMENTS [209]

■ Median percentile Intake (WHO)	3.5-7 mg/day
■ Range (IAEA)	0.1-1.6 mg/day
■ Requirements	Not precisely worked out. A tentative value for adult humans was suggested to be not less than 8 μg Sn/day.

TOXICITY [2,7,200,209]

- Inorganic Sn compounds are relatively non-toxic. Trialkyl substituted compounds are most toxic organo Sn compounds. These may cause:

  – Severe damage to CNS

  – Binding with mitochondria. Inhibition of oxidative phosphorylation.
- Organo Sn compounds have been reported to cause encephalopathy.
- Toxicity may occur following ingestion of contaminated canned food/fruit juices.

  – Nausea, vomiting, diarrhoea

  – Ataxia
- Prolonged exposure to Sn dust causes pneumoconiosis. Toxicity has been reported following exposure to welding fumes.
- Interactions with other contaminants (As, Pb, Sb) may cause anaemia and adversely affect bone mineralisation and cellular functions.
- Tin inhibits hemopoiesis.
- No teratogenic or carcinogenic effects reported. Breast cancer patients showed lower Sn concentrations vs. healthy tissue.
- Earlier staphylococcal infections were treated with Sn. Presence of trialkyl Sn as an impurity caused major poisoning episodes in France.

TITANIUM (Ti)

CATEGORY

Non-essential accumulative ultra-trace element. Some consider it to be a biostimulant/growth enhancer.

DISTRIBUTION IN ECOSYSTEMS [118]

Earth's crust	0.6%
Sea water	1-2 µg/L
Plants	1 mg/kg dry weight

HUMAN BODY [93,193]

Whole body content

Total content in an average adult man (60 kg)	15 mg.

Distribution

Widely distributed in more than 30 human tissues and body fluids including whole blood, erythrocytes, serum, all parts of the gastro-intestinal tract, vital organs, milk, skin, muscles, tooth dentine and enamel, hair and nails. It may accumulate in lungs and lymphatic system.

INTAKE/REQUIREMENTS [118]

Intake	0.3-1.0 mg/day

It is not required for any physiological function.

GUIDELINE VALUES [118]

Occupational Exposure Limit (MAK)	5-10 mg/m^3 dust in air

MEDICINAL USES [15]

Titanium alloys are used in dental amalgams.

TOXICITY [15,81,118]

Ti dioxide, in its pigmentary form, is considered a nuisance dust. These pigments are used as additives to impart whiteners to food items. Contamination may also occur from its uses in cosmetics, dental amalgams, tooth paste and pharmaceuticals. It is corrosive and Ti compounds may cause acid burns. Usage over 6 decades indicates that human body tolerates Ti but there is some experimental evidence for its carcinogenic effects : fibrosarcomas, lymphosarcomas and microscopic lung tumours in rats and mice.

TUNGSTON/WOLFRAM (Wo)

CATEGORY

Non-essential accumulative ultra-trace element.

DISTRIBUTION IN ECOSYSTEMS [118]

Air	< 1.5 μg/m^3
Sea water	0.1 μg/L
Rain water	< 1 μg/L

HUMAN BODY [93,193]

Presence has been reported in whole blood, serum, heart, lungs, bones, skin, tooth enamel and urine.

INTAKE/REQUIREMENTS [209]

Intake	13 μg/day

It is not required for any physiological function.

GUIDELINE VALUES [118]

	W mg/m³ air
Occupational Exposure Limit	
Insoluble compounds	5
Soluble compounds	1

MEDICINAL USES [15]

Dental amalgams

TOXICITY [118,192]

Tungston compounds are not considered a major health hazard in man. Industrial exposure may occur from its uses in tool manufacturing industry. Occupational exposure to W carbide may cause bronchial asthma and progressive interstitial fibrosis. Combination W carbide with Co is reported to cause toxic reaction in lungs. If Co content is greater than 2%, air concentrations at work place should not exceed 0.1 mg/m^3. LD_{50} for W tungstate in rats was found to be 250 μg/kg. Some reports of toxic effects on respiratory system in guinea pigs are also available. Tungstic acid has been used to induce basotemporal epilepsy in cats.

MECHANISM OF TOXICITY [121]

- Gene expression through several signal transduction pathways may be involved in the toxicity and tumorigenicity of Walloys used in military operations.

URANIUM (U)

CATEGORY

Non-essential accumulative ultra-trace element.

DISTRIBUTION IN ECOSYSTEMS [15,172]

AIR	**U ng/m³**
North America	0.2
Europe	0.02
	U μg/m³
Surface air	100
WATER	**U mg/m³**
Sea water	3
Fresh water	0.4
	U μg/l
Drinking water	
Salt Lake City, (USA)	0.67-3.21
Ahmedabad, (India)	22.4
SOIL	**U mg/kg**
Content in surface soil, mean (range)	2 (1-4)

HUMAN BODY [15,93,172]

Whole body content

Total content in average adult man (70 kg)	38 μg

Values as high as 100 - 125 μg have also been reported.

Tissues/body fluids

Blood	**U μg/l**
Whole blood	0.10-0.55
Erythrocytes	0.24

Serum	20
Tissues	**U µg/kg f**
Liver	0.23
Lungs	1.08
Kidneys	0.44
Heart	0.16
Skeleton	0.60
Tracheobronchial lymph node	24.80

ROLE

Uranium has no physiological role in the body.

METABOLISM [172]

Absorption

Absorption occurs through ingestion, inhalation and occasionally through puncture wounds. Gastrointestinal absorption : 1.4%. Inhalatory absorption occurs from air, dust, industrial fumes and cigarette smoking. Puncture wounds constitute an important route of U absorption.

Distribution

Following absorption, it is widely distributed in many tissues and body fluids with highest concentration in tracheobronchial lymph nodes. Content in each organ/tissue is calculated by multiplying the concentration with organ/tissue weight in reference man. The major content is found in skeleton.

Excretion

Excretion occurs in urine, feces and exhaled air.

INTAKE/REQUIREMENTS [172]

	U µg/day
Salt Lake City (USA)	5.67 ± 0.65
Ahmedabad (India)	31.4-59.2

(More water consumed in summer leads to higher intake).

Uranium, being a non-essential element, is not required for man and animals.

GUIDELINE VALUES [15,118]

Occupational exposure limit	:	0.2 mg/m^3 air
Exposure limit for ^{238}U		
Ingestion	:	5×10^5
Inhalation	:	3×10^4
Agricultural soil	:	5 mg/kg dry weight
Limits in drinking water (US-EPA)	:	100 μg/l

TOXICITY [15,81,172,195]

Sources of Exposure/Contamination

From industrial, military and medical uses in:

(*a*) Fission reactors

(*b*) Bomb fuel

(*c*) Armour piercing shells

(*d*) Ship blast and military uses

(*e*) Electron microscopy

(*f*) Radioisotopes

(*g*) Tile glazing etc.

It causes chemical and radiation toxicity.

Signs and Symptoms

- Dermatitis
- Hepatotoxicity
- Nephrotoxicity
- Mutagenic, carcinogenic and teratogenic effects: bone sarcomas, lung cancer, developmental defects, growth retardation and impaired brain function.
- Biochemical changes in blood
- Death may occur following acute exposure.

MECHANISMS OF TOXICITY [15,121]

- Ionizing radiations and mutagenic effects
- Free UO_2^{2+} reacts with renal tubular cells.
- Depleted U, with military applications, was recently shown to activate gene expression through several signal transduction pathways that may be involved in the toxicity and tumorigenicity.

TREATMENT [15,88]

- Chelation using Ca EDTA
- Use of carbonates, citrates and other supportive measures.

VANADIUM (V)

CATEGORY

- Possibly essential ultra-trace element.

DISTRIBUTION IN ECOSYSTEMS [118]

	V ppm Mean (Range)
Soil	66 (49.7-79.0)

PLANT FOODS [118]

	V mg/kg
Cereals	0.08-2.30
Potatoes	0.01-0.02
Fruits	0.008-0.06
Mushrooms	0.001

High content in oils rich in linoleic acid (*e.g.*, Sunflower oil)

ANIMAL FOODS [118]

	V mg/kg
Bovine liver	0.02-0.20
Bovine kidney	0.03-0.12

HUMAN BODY [93,158]

Whole Body Content

- Total number of atoms : 2.4×10^{20}

  Atoms in each cell : 2.4×10^{6}
- 0.3 ppm
- Total content in average adult man (60 kg): 20-25 mg

Distribution

- Presence reported in >39 tissues and body fluids.
- Isotopic studies in rats showed the following order:

  Bones > Kidneys > Liver > Spleen > Intestines > Stomach > Muscles > Testes > Lungs > Brain
- Subcellular distribution in liver was found to be:

  – Nucleus : 43%

  – Mitochondria : 37%

  – Microsomes : 10%

  – Supernatant : 20%

ROLE [118,200]

- Affects (*a*) several enzymes reactions, (*b*) sodium pump, (*c*) redox processes, (*d*) metabolism of carbohydrates, lipids and Fe, (*e*) bone and teeth formation and (*f*) hormonal functions.
- It exerts a catalytic action in the oxidation of phospholipids and catecholamines.
- Activates insulin and elevates its level (?)
- Inhibits (*a*) Coenzyme Q_{10} which is required for electron transport in mitochondria and scavenging of free radicals, (*b*) Cytochrome P_{450}, (*c*) Monoxygenase, (*d*) Methyl transferase, and (*e*) Acetyl coenzyme A.
- Reduces biosynthesis of cholesterol, triglycerides and phospholipids.
- Higher plasma V concentrations have been reported in maniac and depressed patients vs. healthy subjects.

DEFICEINCY [118,209]

Experimental Animals Chicks, Rats

- Abnormal bone development, growth retardation and weight loss.
- Reduced fertility and increased pup mortality.
- Impaired carbohydrate and lipid metabolism.

- Impaired renal function, sodium retention and edema.
- Response of thyroid peroxidase to changing dietary I is affected by V

Man

- Human deficiency has not been reported.
- There is some evidence for role in following conditions. This evidence is not complete.
  - Diabetes (Therapy)
  - Arteriosclerosis (Therapy)
  - Dental caries (Deficiency)
  - Nutritional edema (Deficiency)
  - Maniac Depressive Psychosis (Excess)

METABOLISM [209]

Absorption

- Bulk of orally ingested V remains unabsorbed. Particulate forms are rapidly absorbed from lungs.
- Tracer studies indicated the following absorption times from various routes:

Oral and s/c	:	1 - 6 h
i.p.	:	30 min
intratracheal	:	5 min.

Binding

- V gets mainly bound to transferrin
- Bindings occurs intracellularly in vanadyl (IV) form to the following co-ordinating groups:
  – SH, – OH, – COO–, – SS, – N – $–PO_4$
- Binding in liver cells is associated with high molecular weight proteins.

Excretion

- Bulk of ingested V is unabsorbed and excreted in feces.
- Remaining part is excreted in urine and feces.

INTAKE/REQUIREMENTS [209]

- Average dietary intake : 20 μg/day
- RDA values
  - (*a*) Animals : < 100 μg/kg of diet
  - (*b*) Man : Not worked out. Tentative value suggested for minimum dietary intake was 10 μg/day. Signs of toxicity are observed at intake levels 10 mg/day.

GUIDELINE VALUES [118]

	V mg/m^3
Occupational exposure limit for fumes and dust in air	0.05

MEDICINAL USES [48,66,67,75,76,124,186]

- **Older use:** Anaemias, diabetes, tuberculosis, and as an antiseptic and spirochetocidal agent. With availability of specific and effective drugs, these uses have been abandoned.
- **Investigational stage:** Diammonium-oxy-tartrate vanadate is being investigated for use as a hypo-cholesterolemic and anti-hyperglycemic agent. Use of sodium orthovanadate alone and in combination with some anti-diabetic medicinal plants (*e.g., Momordica charantia* and *Trigonella foenum graecum*) exhibited beneficial effects in diabetes mellitus. Possible use of vanadate as insulin-replacement therapy has been suggested. Several derivatives of V show anti-proliferative activity. Their toxicity must be overcome for therapeutic utility against cancer.

TOXICITY [209]

- ***Oral:*** Chances of poisoning through this route are remote. Gastro-intestinal disturbances and green tongue may occur following excessive V intake.
- ***Inhalation of fumes:*** Causes irritation of respiratory passages and conjunctiva with symptoms of nausea, rhinitis, cough, conjunctivitis, bronchospasms, asthma, chest pain and reduction in vital capacity of lungs.
- ***Carcinogenicity:*** Administration of 5 μg/ml vanadium sulphate in drinking water of mice for life exhibited no carcinogenic action. Excess V exposure was linked to brain tumours in Kuwait.

MECHANISM OF TOXICITY

(*a*) Irritative action of V fumes on respiratory epithelium

(*b*) Release of histamine elicits asthmogenic effects

(*c*) Reduced synthesis of Na^+/K^+ ATPase and vasoconstrictor effects

(*d*) Reduced synthesis of coenzyme A

(*e*) Affects hepatic and SH group enzymes

(*f*) Lowers ascorbic acid levels

(*g*) It is hypothesized that it interferes with sodium pump and causes maniac depressive psychosis

TREATMENT

No specific antidote. Chelation with DTPA and administration of vitamins B and C provides relief.

XENON (Xe)

CATEGORY

Inert gas. Not reported in human body.

YITTRIUM (Y)

CATEGORY

Non-essential accumulative ultra-trace element.

DISTRIBUTION IN ECOSYSTEMS [118]

Earth's crust	3.0 ppm
Soils	2.5-250 ppm
Sea-water (Y^{3+} ions)	0.01-0.3 ppb
Ground water (Y^{3+} ions)	59-73 ppb

Accumulation reported in plants but not in animals.

HUMAN BODY [93,193]

Widely distributed. Presence reported in more than 20 human tissues and body fluids : whole blood, plasma, heart, brain, liver, kidneys, lungs, ovaries, testes, spleen, prostate glands, pancreas, lymph nodes, thymus, thyroid, adrenals, breast, muscles, all parts of the gastro-intestinal tract, aorta, bones and tooth enamel.

ROLE/ESSENTIALITY

No nutritional/physiological role or deficiency syndrome has been reported for this element.

METABOLISM [118]

Absorption

Gastro-intestinal absorption is very poor (about 0.05%). Inhalatory absorption (10-18%) may be more critical. Dermal absorption for ^{90}Y has been demonstrated. Radio-colloidal ^{90}Y is absorbed from intact or injured skin with difficulty. Skin absorption is markedly influenced by pH.

Binding/Metabolism

After absorption it gets bound to gama globulin or albumin in colloidal form and distributed to many tissues and body fluids. Uptake by soft tissues is easy but absorption into bones and bone marrow is slow. Placental barrier is not readily crossed by Y. It has a long biological half-life (about 19 days in respiratory tract). Deposition in lungs occurs in significant quantities. Colloidal Y protein is removed from blood by phagocytes in the reticulo-endothelial system and liver.

Excretion

Excretion occurs in urine and feces. Excretion via urine is very slow (about 40% in a week). It is also secreted in milk and colostrum is reported to have high Y content.

GUIDELINE VALUES 118

Occupational Exposure Limit	Y mg/m^3
USSR	2
Germany	5
USA	5

MEDICINAL USES 79

^{90}Y has been used for chemical synovectomy as a substitute for surgical operation in cases of arthritis.

TOXICITY 118

Though few data are available, Y is generally considered to have low toxicity. Sources of contamination are from its use in ceremic industry, electronics, colour television, data processing equipment, superconductors and nuclear reactors. Inhalatory exposure to Y containing dust is more critical vs. its oral uptake. Toxic effects are attributed to its ability to displace Ca^{2+} ions and interfere with functions of calmodulin. Y^{3+} ions have higher affinity for calmodulin binding sites than Ca^{2+}. This causes increase in phosphodiestrase activity, disrupts cAMP-dependent processes, neuron activity, secretary processes (hormones, transmitters and enzymes), calcification effects and detoxification mechanisms. It is reported to decrease immune resistance and produce lung granulomas consisting of crystalline Y oxide deposits and cellular elements. Carcinogenesis following oral exposure of mice (5 ppm for life) is doubtful; some reports revealed no tumours after 3 generation of feeding Y oxide.

YTTERBIUM (Yb)

CATEGORY

Non-essential accumulative ultra-trace element.

DISTRIBUTION IN ECOSYSTEMS 118

Earth's crust	3 ppm

HUMAN BODY [93,193]

Presence reported in whole blood, serum, diaphragm and tooth enamel.

ZINC (Zn)

CATEGORY

Essential trace element.

DISTRIBUTION IN ECOSYSTEM [15,118]

AIR	**Zn ng/m³**
Remote Areas (Greenland)	18-41
North America	500
Europe	1,200
North India (Ludhiana, Chandigarh)	241-8549
WATER	**Zn mg/m³**
Sea water	5
Fresh water	15

Ground water: Zn may get mobilized into it from the soil under acidic conditions. Consumption and use of such water should be restricted to protect public health.

SOIL	**Zn mg/kg**
Mean (Range)	60 (15-220)

PLANTS [118]

Bioaccumulation Index (Plant : Soil ratio)	1 to 10
Concentration at which no sensitivity develops in immature plants	100-400 mg/kg dry matter
Food Plants	**Zn mg/kgf**
Cereals	13-41
Potatoes	8.51
Vegetables	4.51
Fruits	1.66
Mushrooms	9.7-280
Tea	35.0
Coffee	6.7

ANIMAL FOODS [118]

Zinc content is more in non-vegetation diet vs. vegetarian diet. Organ meats and oyesters are rich in Zn content.

	Zn mg/kgf
Milk	3.5
Meat	20-60
Liver	100-150
Kidney	50-100
Fish	1.5
Oyesters	100-200 (upto 2g in some varieties)

HUMAN BODY [9,93,158,200,209]

Whole Body Content

- 1500 atoms per billion atoms
- 30 mg/kg of fat-free tissues
- 33 ppm
- Content in an average adult man (60 kg) : approx. 2.3 g

Distribution

- Widely distributed in >50 tissues and body fluids including all vital organs.
- It is a constituent of >200 bioproteins/enzymes and is known to be required for about 100 mammalian enzymes.
- **Blood**

	Zn mg/L
Erythrocytes	14.2 (7.6-16.1)
Plasma	1.14 (0.79-1.70)
Serum	1.15 (0.67-1.83)

- **Tissues**

  Highest tissue concentrations are reported in prostate, liver, muscles, kidneys, and brain. While total body Zn is approximately half the total body Fe, in the brain the values are almost equal.

- **Homeostasis :** Redistribution of Zn between extracellular and intracellular compartments by release of a leucocyte endogenous mediator (LEM) which is a key factor in Zn homeostasis during infection.

ROLE/ESSENTIALITY [58,70,118,200,209]

■ Zinc has important role in various **enzymatic reactions**. Some examples are given below:

Constituent of Enzyme	Consequences of Absence/Deficiency
Alkaline phosphatase	Whole energy metabolism compromised
Alcohol dehydrogenase	Alcohol intoxication
Carbonic anhydrase	Acidosis
Glutathione dehydrogenase	Transamination reactions stopped
Lactate dehydrogenase	Lactate accumulation, muscular acidosis and fatigue.
Superoxide dismutase	Cell destruction by free radicals.

■ **Protein synthesis** (including nuclear proteins : RNA, DNA)

■ **Replication, transcription and translation** of genetic material.

■ **Hormonal function** : pituitary, insulin, reproductive hormones.

■ By above mechanisms, it exerts effect on:

(*a*) growth

(*b*) reproduction

(*c*) wound healing/healthy skin

(*d*) maintenance of membrane structure and function

(*e*) protection against free-radical damage

(*f*) immune function etc.

■ **Zinc fingers**

DEFICIENCY [50,118,144,191,200,209]

■ Deficiency of Zn, under normal condition, is unlikely. Conditioned Zn deficiency/loss may occur in following cases:

(*a*) Alcoholics

(*b*) Patients on total parenteral nutrition

(*c*) Infections

(*d*) Burns

(*e*) Diabetes

(*f*) Renal disease/Dialysis therapy/Use of diuretics

(*g*) Liver disease

(*h*) Chronic blood loss

(*i*) Sickle-cell anaemia

(*j*) Use of chelating agents etc.

- **Marginal Zn deficiency** states are difficult to detect. These may be manifested by non-specific clinical features *e.g.* (*a*) growth retardation/dwarfism, (*b*) rough skin, (*c*) poor appetite, (*d*) mental lethargy, (*e*) slow healing of wounds, (*f*) impaired immune function, (*g*) susceptibility to infections, (*h*) thyroid dysfunction, (*i*) hepatosplenomegaly, (*j*) hypogonadism etc.

- **Seminal plasma** of normospermic males contains more Zn vs. that in Oligospermic and azoospermic subjects.

- **Diagnosis :** Wide variations in baseline values (serum, plasma and hair Zn levels) are reported. The following are considered good indices/diagnostic features for Zn deficiency:

  (*a*) Dysomia (impaired taste)

  (*b*) Delayed dark adaptation

  (*c*) Activities of Zn-binding proteins

- **Zn Deficiency Diseases**

  (*a*) *Acrodermatitis Enteropathica:* It is an autosomal recessively inherited genetic Zn deficiency disease manifested mainly by gastrointestinal symptoms and skin lesions. The latter include alopecia, paronychia, bullous pustular dermatitis (more in oral, anal and genital areas and on extremities). Other symptoms include nutritional disturbances, diarrhoea, blepharitis, conjunctivitis, depressed mood and growth failure.

  (*b*) *Male hypogonadism:* It was reported in Iranian males. Besides inhibitory effect on gonads and reproductive function, the deficiency was manifested by rough skin, anemia, lethargy and dwarfism. Both the diseases responded to Zn supplementation.

- **Effects on developing fetus:** CNS and skeletal abnormalities and low birth weights.

METABOLISM [15,209]

- ***Site:*** Absorption of orally-ingested Zn mainly takes place from small intestines (particularly distal duodenum and proximal part of jejunum).
- ***Extent:*** There is considerable variation for extent of oral absorption. It is reported to be 20-80% from food and 43-66% from drinking water.
- ***Factors Affecting Absorption:***
  - (*a*) Type of compound: oxide and free metal are well absorbed, sulphate and mixed oxides (with Zn and Mn) are poorly absorbed.
  - (*b*) Requirement/Demand: Absorption is better in deficiency states.
  - (*c*) Pathological conditions: Absorption is depressed,
  - (*d*) Food items: While high phytate, fibre, soya protein, Cd, Ca, Cu elicit an inhibitory effect, red wine (no other alcoholic beverage), some amino acids *e.g.*, histidine enhance absorption. Better Zn availability is reported from mother's milk vs. cow milk.
- ***Controls:*** Absorption of Zn is through a saturable carrier-mediated process under homeostatic control by metallothionein.

Binding/Metabolism

- **Binding:** occurs with plasma proteins: albumin, α-2 macroglobulin and transferrin.
- **Distribution Turnover:** It is distributed in bound form to all tissues and body fluids. It crosses both the blood-brain and placental barriers. While the uptake and turnover rate of Zn is rapid for some vital organs *e.g.*, liver, kidney, pancreas and spleen, it is poor for bones and central nervous system where it is retained for longer time in bound form.

Excretion

- **Two Phase Process:** First phase (10-20%) is relatively rapid with a median half life of 7 to 14 days. Second phase (80%) is slow and has a median half life of 160 to 500 days.
- **Route:** Bulk of the ingested Zn (70-80%, 5-10 mg/day) is excreted in feces, bile and pancreatic juice, urinary excretion is low (0.4-0.6 mg/day). There may be substantial excretion through sweat in hot weather (upto 3 mg/day).

INTAKE/REQUIREMENTS [118,129,209]

Intake	Zn mg/day
■ Intake in industrialized countries in populations on diets high in fat, refined sugar and animal protein.	10-12

- United Kingdom (survey on 2100 adults, values in mean ± SD) — 9.7 ± 3.3

Recommended Dietary Allowances (RDA)

	Zn mg/day
Infants upto 6 months	3
6 months to 1 year	5
Children 1 to 10 years	10
Adults	15
Pregnant women	20
Lactating women	25

Studies from Egypt, Kenya and Mexico revealed significant positive correlation between intake of animal source food and growth, cognitive development and physical activity in school children.

GUIDELINE VALUES

■ Drinking water (India)	
Permissible	5 mg/l
Excessive	15 mg/l
■ Occupational Exposure Level (OEL, for 40-h work week)	1 - 5 mg/m^3
■ Biological Exposure Limit	
Blood	10 μg/L
Hair	150-200 μg/g
■ Maximum Tolerable Intake (WHO)	0.3-1 mg/kg/day
■ Composted sewage sludge	300 mg/kg

MEDICINAL USES 28,31,32,44,53,55,86,105,118,119,129,141,146,195,200,213

- **Deficiency States:**
  - Acrodermatitis Enteropathica
  - Male Hypogonadism/Infertility
- **Miscellaneous Systemic Uses:** Some clinical studies have shown beneficial effects in following diseases:
  - Acute lymphocytic leukemia
  - Age-related macular degeneration
  - Alcoholic cirrhosis

- Arteriosclerosis
- Arthritis
- Indian childhood cirrhosis
- Cataract
- Chronic hepatitis
- Common cold
- Complications of pregnancy/still births: The incidence is reduced following Zn treatment.
- Diarrhoea
- Pneumonia
- Root-end dental filling
- Shigellosis

■ **Local/External Uses:** Preparations of Zn, with antiseptic and astringent properties, are used in skin and eye diseases, wounds, burns etc.

- Zn oxide is used in dusting powders, ointments, lotions, adhesive tape.
- Zn chloride and acetate are incorporated in astringent solutions.
- Other Zn compounds used for medicinal purposes include stearate, oleate, permangnate etc.

Metal contamination of soils and crops from a Pb/Zn mine spill in Southern China has recently been reported. Consumption of such crops may be hazardous to human health. Leafy vegetables in soil irrigated with sewage sludge and effluent may pose similar danger.

TOXICITY [15,27,50,69,86,107,118,128,183]

Sources of Exposure

galvanized/Zn plated containers may accumulate concentrations upto 2 g/L.

Though Zn is a relatively non-toxic metal vs. As, Cd, Pb, Sb etc, toxicity may occur from exposure in industrial workers and common usage in:

(*a*) Galvanizing of iron and steel for corrosion protection. Acidic fruit juices stored in
(*b*) Alloys
(*c*) Welding
(*d*) Vulcanizing of rubber
(*e*) Ryan glass
(*f*) Enamel and Plastics
(*g*) Paints

(*h*) TV tubes
(*i*) Fertilizers
(*j*) Photocopying paper
(*k*) Medicines and cosmetics etc.

Symptoms

Acute toxicity is manifested by nausea vomiting, colic, diarrhoea, severe anaemia cramps, fever, renal failure and fatal shock. Industrial exposure to fumes cause **Metal Fume Fever**, with predominantly pulmonary symptoms fever, chills and gastroenteritis.

SYSTEMIC EFFECTS

1. ***Liver:*** Pathogenesis is more often associated with deficiency rather than excess of Zn. Low plasma/serum Zn levels have been reported in infective hepatitis, chronic active hepatitis, hepatosplenomegaly, alcoholic cirrhosis, Hodgkin's disease and Wilson's disease. Hair and liver Zn concentrations were found to be low in Indian childhood cirrhosis. Urinary Zn excretion increased in cases of cirrhosis and infective hepatitis. The values returned to normal levels when the disease subsided. Zinc is a major component of biliary calculi.
2. ***Kidney:*** Uremia patients exhibited decrease in plasma/serum Zn levels. Urinary Zn excretion is markedly increased in cases of nephrosis and albiuminurea (1.0 to 3.8 mg/day) vs. normal healthy subjects (0.1 to 0.7 mg/day). Nephrotic kidney is not able to provide an effective barrier to bound Zn in plasma and, therefore, porphyrinuria is a frequently observed symptom in occupationally exposed persons.
3. ***Central nervous system:*** Brain and choroid plexus of retina are rich in Zn content. Deficiency of this element during pregnancy and lactation is linked to congenital abnormalities. Low learning ability, apathy, lethargy, mood, fluctuations and psychotic behaviour are associated with low Zn status. High CSF concentrations were observed in patients with damaged blood-brain barrier, subarachnoid hemorrhage and malignant tumours. Ex-heroin addicts and untreated epilepsy patients had lower CSF Zn concentrations vs. normal healthy subjects.
4. ***Cardiovascular system:*** Effects are known for low Zn status rather than for its excess. Atherosclerosis and myocardial infarction are associated with decrease in hair and plasma Zn levels. These reports have both diagnostic (alterations in plasma Zn during first 3 days in myocardial infarction) and therapeutic (Zn therapy in atherosclerosis) implications.
5. ***Respiratory system:*** Inhalatory exposure to Zn oxide fumes (particle size < 1 mμ) may cause metal fume fever. Low serum Zn levels were reported in bronchial carcinoma and tuberculosis.

6. ***Skin:*** Effects are related to deficiency states (**Acrodermatitis enteropathica**) and medicinal uses discussed in other sections. In many infectious diseases (including leprosy) urinary excretion of Zn increases resulting in depleted serum Zn levels.

7. ***Reproductive system:***

   (*a*) *Pregnancy and lactation:* Serum Zn levels get depleted with increased demand; values < 50 μg/L indicate inadequate Zn status. Deficiency states are associated with higher incidence of maternal (delayed labour, necessity for surgical interventions for delivery) and fetal (low birth weights) complications. Marked decline in plasma Zn levels has been reported in cases with hypertension, toxaemia of pregnancy and congenital defects. White therapeutic supplementation has beneficial results, some reports of premature deliveries and still births call for a cautious approach. Indiscriminate Zn supplements (without establishing deficient status) should, therefore, be avoided.

   (*b*) *Fertility and sterility :* Deficiency causes **Male hypogonadism**, reduced sperm count, viability and motility, chronic prostato-vesiculitis, secretary dysfunction and infertility. Adverse effects on testicular function are reversed by Zn supplementation. Zn chloride (500 ppm in drinking water) was shown to protect male mice against chronic potassium chromate (150 ppm in drinking water) - induced testicular injury.

8. ***Immune function:*** Deficiency states impair cellular and humoral immunity in man and animals. Exposure to Zn causes an increase in bone marrow precursor cells but exerts an inhibitory action on proliferation of B-lymphocytes and T-dependent antibody response. Therapy in people (>70 years) has been reported to increase total lymphocyte count, serum immunoglobulin levels and delayed type hypersensitivity. Convincing evidence for the so called 'immune boosting' supplements in preventing exercise-induced immune impairment in sportsmen is currently lacking. It is mildly mitogenic and immunotoxic in large doses. Toxic doses inhibit lymphocyte proliferation response to phytoheme-agglutinin, chemotactic migration and phygocytic activity. The susceptibility to infection is increased. Immune complex reaction to inhaled Zn oxide fumes causes metal fume fever.

9. ***Mutagenicity/Carcinogenicity:*** Hypoparathyroidism, deafness and renal dysplasia (HDR) syndrome is an autosomal dominant disorder caused by mutations of the dual Zn finger transcription factor, GATA-3. Mutations in GATA-1 in its cofactor FOG-1 have been linked to thrombocytopenia and thalassemia. Significantly low blood/serum Zn concentrations have been reported in many tumours *e.g.*, bronchial and prostatic carcinoma, multiple myeloma, lymphoma, Hodgkin's disease, chronic lymphocytic leukemia etc. There is no evidence for the carcinogenic effects of Zn except with Zn chromate (like other chromates). The metal is,

however, needed for cellular proliferation of existing tumours. Therapeutic use of colloidal radioactive ^{63}Zn has been reported for irradiation of serous cavities (lungs, bladder, peritoneal cavities) and in chemosurgery (cautery) of malignant tumours.

10. ***Teratogenic effects:*** No reports are available for such effects due to excess of Zn; teratogenic effects have been demonstrated in Zn deficient experimental animals and suspected in humans.

MECHANISM OF TOXICITY [15,118]

- Impaired immune function: Inhibitory effect on lymphocyte proliferation, chemotaxis and phagocytic activity.
- Irritative/corrosive actions.

TREATMENT [15,118]

- **Chelation therapy:** Di-sodium CaEDTA and unithiol.
- **Supportive measures:** Alkaline inhalations, glucose, vitamin C, tea/coffee, cardiac drugs, antibiotics etc. according to the symptomatic demand.

ZIRCONIUM (Zr)

CATEGORY

Non-essential accumulative trace element.

DISTRIBUTION IN ECOSYSTEMS [118]

Earth's crust	150-300 ppm
Fresh	0.002 - 0.02 ppm
Sea water	0.02 - 0.5 ppb
Plants	0.3 - 2 ppm dry weight

HUMAN BODY [15,93,118,193]

Total content in average adult man (60 kg)	300 mg

Presence has been reported in 24 human tissues and body fluids : whole blood, erythrocytes, serum, bones, brain, breast, gall bladder, stomach, jejunum, colon, hair, heart, kidney, liver, lungs, lymph nodes, skeletal muscles, nails, ovary, pancreas, spleen, testes, tooth enamel and urine.

MEDICINAL USES [15,81]

It is used in cosmetics for its antiperspirant and deodorant properties. The element is useful in the treatment of dermatitis due to poisoning and *Rhus* plants.

GUIDELINE VALUES [118]

Occupational Exposure Limit (MAK)	5 mg/m^3 air
Agricultural soil	300 mg/kg day weight

TOXICITY [81,118]

Use of Zr containing cosmetics may cause **Axillary granuloma** and should, therefore, be discouraged. While Zr is generally considered to be of low toxicity, chronic inhalatory exposure is reported to cause lung disease and cancer. The metal may contribute to the local effects of ceramic implants/fixed prosthesis.

3

DISEASES/SYNDROMES

3.1 DISEASES DUE TO ELEMENTAL DEFICIENCIES	
ELEMENT	*DISEASE/ SYNDROME*
Calcium	Rickets, Osteomalacia, Osteoporosis, Clotting defects
Chromium (Glucose Tolerance Factor)	Diabetes mellitus
Cobalt (Cobalamine/Vitamin B_{12})	Pernicious anemia
Copper	Hypochromic microcytic anemia Menke's kinky hair syndrome
Fluorine	Dental caries
Iodine	Myxedematous cretinism Goitre Hypothyroidism Sterility
Iron	Hypochromic microcytic anemia Dwarfism Fatigue Plummer Vinson syndrome Sidropenic dysphagia
Magnesium	Acute pancreatitis Idiopathic epilepsy
Manganese	Hyperplasia of pancreas Skeletal abnormalities
Oxygen	Hypoxia Cyanosis Asthma Respiratory failure
Phsophorous	Osteomalacia Osteoporosis

Potassium	Diabetic acidosis Renal insufficiency/edema Hyperfunction of adrenal cortex Muscular weakness
Selenium	Keshan's disease Kaschin Beck disease
Silicon	Atherosclerosis Aging
Sodium	Dehydration Hypovolemic shock Muscle cramps
Sulphur	Detoxification mechanisms compromised
Vanadium	Disturbed Iron and Lipid metabolism
Zinc	Acrodermatitis enteropathica Male hypogonadism

3.2 DISEASES ASSOCIATED WITH OVEREXPOSURE/TOXICITY OF ELEMENTS

ELEMENT	*DISEASE/ SYNDROME*
Aluminium	Dialysis dementia Dialysis osteodystrophy Alzheimer's disease
Arsenic	Black foot disease/Dry gangrene Rain drop rash Peripheral neuropathy Squamous cell carcinoma
Beryllium	Pulmonary granulomatosis
Cadmium	Itai Itai disease
Cobalt	Polycythemia
Copper	Grape Garden Sprayer's disease Indian childhood cirrhosis Schizophrenia (?) Wilson's disease
Fluorine	Mottled teeth/ weak enamel Knock knee
Gold	Aplastic anemia Mucocutaneous reactions Thrombocytopenia
Iodine	Thyrotoxicosis Exophthalmic goitre
Iron	Hemochromatosis Sideroblastic anemia Porphyria cutanea tarda Susceptibility to infections and cancer
Lead	Encephalopathy Palsy Learning disability Mental retardation Wrist and foot drop Anemia with reticulocytosis
Manganese	Parkinson's disease-like syndrome Sclerosis amyotrophic lateralis
Mercury	Minamata disease Pink disease

Molybdenum	Gout
Nickel	Allergic contact dermatitis Pneumonia
Osmium	Insomnia Headache Halo effects on vision
Platinum	Allergic dermatitis Asthma Platinosis: irritation of skin and mucus membranes of eyes and respiratory tract.
Radium	Radiation effects Cancer
Selenium	Endemic human selenosis reported in China with symptoms of garlic-like odour in breath, bad teeth, icteroid skin, dermatitis, hair loss, gastro-intestinal disturbances, inflammation of mucus membranes, loss of appetite, headache, heartburn, convulsions, paralysis etc.
Silicon	Silicosis with TB
Silver	Blue pigmentation of elastic fibres in skin, respiratory tract and eyes
Sodium	Hypertension Edema Cardiac failure
Tellurium	Suppression of sweating Gastro-intestinal and CNS disturbances
Tin	Benign pneumoconiasis
Uranium	Radiation hazard/ Cancer Renal damage
Vanadium	Irritative respiratory syndrome
Zinc	Metal fume fever
Zirconium	Axillary granuloma

3.3 CLINICAL APPLICATIONS OF ELEMENTS

ELEMENT	DIAGNOSTIC/THERAPEUTIC USE
Aluminium	(*i*) Antacid (*ii*) Antiperspirant (*iii*) Treatment of fluorosis (*iv*) To reduce phosphate absorption in uremia patients.
Antimony	(*i*) Treatment of helminth infections: – Leishmaniasis – Trypanosomiasis – Schistosmiasis – Filariasis (*ii*) Component of traditional Indian eye cosmetics: *Surma* and *Kajal* (*iii*) Potential value against AIDS virus using Ammonium-5-tungstate-2-antimoniate, a reverse transkriptase inhibitor.
Arsenic	(*i*) Under investigation for anti-cancer effects (*ii*) Calcined As preparations (Ayurvedic and Unani) used for general and nervine tonic, aphrodisiac, anti-rheumatic, anti-arrhythmic and anti-diabetic effects in the Indian sub-continent.
Barium	Contrast media for X-ray
Bismuth	(*i*) Contrast media for X-ray (*ii*) Bi-subcitrate for the treatment of gastric ulcers (*iii*) Bi-oxide and sulphate used in cosmetics
Boron	(*i*) Boric acid is antiseptic, 3% solution used for wounds and warm solution used for washing eyes. (*ii*) Sodium tetraborate (Borax) is claimed to be useful in rheumatoid arthritis.
Cadmium	Cd sulphide (1% suspension) is applied in cases of seborrhoeic dermatitis.

Calcium	Supplements in cases of deficiency or increased demand: (*i*) Pregnancy (*ii*) Growing children (*iii*) Fractures (*iv*) Rickets (*v*) Osteoporosis
Carbon	Activated charcoal is used as adsorbent in cases of poisoning.
Chlorine	(*i*) Germicidal. Used for purification of water (*ii*) Parentral nutrition : i.v. saline, dextrose saline using Na, K or NH_4 salts
Chromium	(*i*) Diabetes mellitus (?). Alterations in urinary Cr values are important because these represent GTF stores of the body (*ii*) Nervine tonic (?)
Cobalt	As cobalamine (Vitamin B_{12}) in pernicious anaemia.
Copper	(*i*) Insecticides, pesticides, fungicides. (*ii*) Intra-uterine contraceptive devices (IUCD) (*iii*) Alterations in serum Cu for first 7 days in the diagnosis of myocardial infarction. Hepatic and urinary Cu levels are markedly elevated in prolonged choleostasis, chronic biliary cirrhosis and Wilson's disease. (*iv*) Traditional use of Cu bracelets for benefit in Arthritis and Cardiovascular diseases (?)
Germanium	Anti-tumour effects
Gold	Treatment of rheumatoid arthritis
Indium	(*i*) Diagnostic use of ^{111}In to localize malignant and inflammatory lesions (*ii*) Oxide is used for organ scanning and for the treatment of hepatic tumours.
Iodine	(*i*) Germicidal application for abrasions, wounds : tincture iodine, iodine lotion. (*ii*) Counter-irritant ointments to treat muscular pain (*iii*) Contrast media for X-ray (*iv*) Treatment of goitre.
Iron	Supplements in deficiency states (anemia) and increased demand (pregnancy, hemorrhage).
Lanthanum	(*i*) Therapeutic use in arthritis (*ii*) Potential value as an anti-cancer agent needs to be explored.

Lead	Cosmetic uses (*i*) carbonate is depitatory (*ii*) acetate is used in hair dyes (*iii*) component of traditional Indian eye cosmetics *Surma* and *Kajal.*
Lithium	Psychiatric medicine: Prophylaxis and treatment of Maniac depressive psychosis (MDP)
Magnesium	(*i*) Mg salts are antacid and $MgSO_4$ is used as a purgative agent. (*ii*) Therapeutic value in cardiovascular diseases: – Hypertension – Stroke – Congestive heart failure – Arrhythmias – Ischemic heart disease – Myocardial infarction (*iii*) Analysis of serum Mg levels for diagnosis of amoebic liver abscess. (*iv*) Semen Mg analysis is useful in male infertility
Manganese	Treatment of Diabetes mellitus (?)
Mercury	(*i*) External uses as an antiseptic, fungicidal and parasiticidal agent. Not used internally in modern medicine. (*ii*) Calcined Ayurvedic mercury preparations *Siddh Makardhwaja* and *Kajjali* are claimed to be therapeutically useful in varied diseases without causing toxicity (?)
Molybdenum	(*i*) Deficiency of xanthine dehydrogenase and sulphite oxidase. (*ii*) Tetrathiomolybdate has been used in cases of Cu toxicity and as an alternative to penicillamine in Wilson's disease.
Oxygen	(*i*) Hypoxia, shock, depressive states, poisoning, drowning. (*ii*) High altitude climbing and diving operations (*iii*) Oxygenated water has been used to treat gastric ulcers.
Phosphorus	(*i*) Rodenticide (*ii*) Smoke screen in war (*iii*) Nervine tonic (?) (*iv*) ^{35}P has been used in cases of Polycythemia vera and Granulocytic leukemia. (*v*) Diagnostic uses in bone disorders, liver disease, and metastatic carcinoma of prostate gland.
Platinum	(*i*) Cis-platinum compounds are used for the chemotherapy of cancer and for antibacterial and antiviral effects. (*ii*) Pt alloys are used in dental amalgams.

Potassium	(*i*) To control cardiac manifestations of Digitalis poisoning (*ii*) Idiopathic therapy with KI in childhood asthma (*iii*) Insulin-dextrose infusion in Angina pectoris (*iv*) K-permanganate is germicidal, citrate is antacid and sodium tartrate is emetic (*v*) Loss associated with diuretics (*vi*) Myoaesthania gravis
Selenium	(*i*) Keshan's Disease (*ii*) Therapeutic value reported in many diseases including atherosclerosis, congestive heart failure, arthritis, viral hepatitis, kwashiorkor, cancer and for reduction of side effects of anti-cancer drugs Cisplantin and Adriamycin without affecting their anticancer activity. (*iii*) SeS useful in seborrhoeic dermatitis and as an anti-dandruff agent in shampoos.
Silicon	(*i*) Potential for therapeutic utility in atherosclerosis needs to be explored. (*ii*) Protective effect shown in cases of simple myopia in children.
Silver	(*i*) Topical use for the treatment of burns, wounds and sepsis. (*ii*) Cautery by $AgNO_3$ to remove warts and moles. (*iii*) Silver is not used internally in modern medicine. Calcined Ag preparations are, however, used in Ayurveda and Unani medicine for varied effects including tonic (general, nervine, cardiac and sexual), rejuvenating effects and claimed utility in bronchitis, asthma, tuberculosis, neuropsychiatric disorders and sexual weakness.
Sodium	(*i*) Oral rehydration fluid in cases of diarrhoea, dysentery and dehydration. (*ii*) Parentral nutrition for fluid replacement using normal saline or dextrose saline.
Strontium	(*i*) Radiotherapy with ^{90}Sr for palliative effect in bone sarcoma, eyelid melanoma and mycosis fungoides. (*ii*) Sr bromide in leprosy (*iii*) Limited use as an adjuvant to Ca for remineralisation of bones in cases of osteoporosis and tooth decay.
Sulphur	(*i*) Topical use for antiseptic and parasiticidal effects in cases of acne, boils, scabies, itching, dermatitis, eczema and leprosy. It is used in the form of ointments, lotions and dusting powders.

	(*ii*) Germicidal fumigant. (*iii*) Chemical weapon of war
Tantalum	*Diagnostic uses:* (*i*) Better visibility vs. Ba and I as contrast medium for X ray. (*ii*) Bronchography (*iii*) Detection of occult cancer (*iv*) Blood-pool imaging (*v*) Radio-opaque biomarker (*vi*) Determination of clearance time in patients with chronic obstructive pulmonary disease. *Other uses:* (*i*) Surgical implants (*ii*) Ophthalmic surgery
Tellurium	Treatment of *Seuborrboea capitis*
Thallium	(*i*) Pesticide/rodenticide
	(*ii*) Ringworm (*iii*) Depilatory agent
Thorium	Superficial *Capillary naevus*
Tin	(*i*) Tapeworm infestation (*ii*) Sn coating of brass/copper utensils is reported to prevent Indian childhood cirrhosis.
Titanium	Skin diseases
Tungston	Dental amalgams
Vanadium	Diammonium-oxy-tartrate-vanadate in cases of hyper-cholesterolemia (?)
Yttrium	Chemical synovectomy using ^{90}Y in arthritis.
Zinc	(*i*) Deficiency states : Acrodermatitis enteropathica Male hypogonadism Infertility (*ii*) Systemic use also reported in complications of pregnancy, still births, atherosclerosis, arthritis, alcoholic cirrhosis, Indian childhood cirrhosis, common cold, gastric ulcers, ulcerative colitis etc (?) (*iii*) Topical use of antiseptic and astringent effects in cases skin and eye diseases, burns and wounds.
Zirconium	(*i*) Used in cosmetics for anti-perspirant and deodorant effects. (*ii*) Treatment of dermatitis due to poisoning and *Rhus* plants.

3.4 INDEX OF DISEASES/SYNDROMES

Constriction of visual field	150
Contraception	78,79,81,251
Contracted kidney	122
Contact dermatitis	34,48,67,168,249
Convulsions	25,54,56,72,130,133,139,196,203,217,249
Cornea, dimming of	173
Coronary occlusion	138,143
Cortical blindness	123,150,174
Corhyza	26,178
Cough	26,34,43,50,152,168,230
Cretinism	104,246
Cyanosis	71,72,168,210,214,246
Cystic fibrosis	191
Cystic tumours	18,25
Cytotoxicity	89,90,94
Dandruff	194,196,253
Deaf-mutism	104
Deafness	72
Dehydration	60,94,205,206,217,247
Delayed estrus	165
Delirium	43,130,168,217
Dementia	43
Demyelination	122,124,176
Dental amalgams	202,222,223,252,254
Dental caries	85,86,159,206,208,246
Depigmentation of hair	161
Depressed phagocytosis	35,113
Depression	181,228,252
Dermatitis	34,48,67,168,178,195,196,210,226,236,249,253

4

REFERENCES

1. ANKE M, BAUMANN W, BRAUNLICH H (1983): *4 Spurenelement Symposium*, Karl-Marx Universitat, Leipzig and Fredrich-Schiller Universitat, Jena.
2. ANKE M, KRAUSE H, GROPPEL B (1987): The effect of arsenic deficiency on growth, reproduction, life expectancy and disease symptoms in animals. In: *Proceedings of Trace Substances in Environmental Health* (Ed.: Hemphill DD), vol. 21, pp. 553-60, University of Missouri, Columbia.
3. ANKE M, SCHNEIDER HJ, BRUCKNER C (1980): *3 Spurenelement Symposium: Nickel*, Karl-Marx Universitat, Leipzig and Fredrich-Schiller Universitat, Jena.
4. ANKE, M, SCHNEIDER HJ, BRUCKNER C (1980): *3 Spurenelement Symposium: Arsen*, Karl-Marx Universitat, Leipzig and Fredrich-Schiller Universitat, Jena.
5. ANONYMOUS (1981): *National Formulary of Unani Medicine*, Part-I, pp. 65-78, Central Council for Research in Unani Medicine, Ministry of Health and Family Welfare, Government of India, New Delhi.
6. ANONYMOUS (1985): *IRPTC 63: Beryllium*, UN Environment Programme, Centre of International Projects, GKNT, Moscow.
7. ANONYMOUS (1985): *Ramington's Practice of Pharmacy*, ED 17, pp. 1030-1031, Mac Publising Co., Easton, Pennsylvania.
8. ANONYMOUS (1987): *Hartal Bhasma*, In: *Pharmacopoeal Standards of Ayurvedic Formulations, Ayurvedic Formulary of India*, Part-I, 18:22, p. 43, Central Council for Research in Ayurveda and Siddha, Ministry of Health and Family Welfare, Government of India, New Delhi.
9. ANONYMOUS (1990): *Environmental Health Criteria 160: Beryllium*, World Health Organization, Geneva.
10. ANONYMOUS (2004): *A Scientific Review: The Role of Chromium in Insulin Resistance*. Diabetes Educ, **Suppl.**, 2-14.
11. ARNOLD SM, LYNN TV, VERBUGGE LA, MIDDAUGH JP (2005): Human biomonitoring to optimize fish consumption advice: reducing uncertainty when evaluating benefits and risks. *Amer J. Publ. Hlth*, **95(3)**, 393-97.
12. ARORA RB, VOHORA SB, KHAN MSY (1984): *Proceedings of the First International Conference on Elements in Health and Disease*, Institute of History of Medicine and Medical Research, New Delhi.
13. ARVIDSON B (1999): Axonal transport and neurotoxic metals. In: *New Aspects of Trace Element Research* (Eds.: Abdulla M, Bost M, Gamon S, Arnaud P, Chazot G), pp. 123-27, Smith-Gordon, London, Nishimura, Tokyo.

14. ASIMOV I (1962): *Marvels of Science*, Ed. 1, pp. 31-34, Collier Books, New York.

15. ATHAR M, VOHORA SB (1995): *Heavy Metals and Environment*, New Age International Publishers Ltd./Wiley Eastern Ltd., New Delhi.

16. AUGER N, KOFMAN O, KOSTSKY T, ARMSTRONG R (2005): Low-level methylmercury exposure as a risk factor for neurologic abnormalities in adults. *Neurotoxicology*, **26(2)**, 149-57.

17. AYESHA (1999). Neuropsychopharmacological and adaptogenic studies on indigenous silver preparations. *Ph.D. Thesis (Toxicology)*, Jamia Hamdard, New Delhi.

18. AYESHA N, BAJAJ S, VOHORA D, VOHORA SB (2000): Effect of calcined gold and silver preparations on experimental models of epilepsy. *Indian J., Toxicol.,* **7(1)**, 11-17.

19. AYESHA, KHANNA T, SIVARAMAN R, VOHORA SB (1997): Analgesic activity of silver preparations used in Indian systems of medicine. *Indian J. Pharmacol.,* **29**, 393-98.

20. AYESHA, KHANNA T, VOHORA SB (1999): Silver preparations used in Indian systems of medicine: Neuropsychobehavioural effects. *Indian J. Pharmacol.*, **31**, 214-22.

21. BAHRAMI AR, MAHJUB H (2003): Comparative study of lung function in Iranian factory workers exposed to silica dust. *East Mediter, Health J.*, **9(3)**, 390-98.

22. BAJAJ S (1999). Neuropsychopharmacological and Immunomodulatory studies on Gold preparations used in Indian systems of medicine. *Ph.D. Thesis (Toxicology)*, Jamia Hamdard, New Delhi.

23. BAJAJ S, AHMAD I, FATIMA M, RAISUDDIN S, VOHORA SB (1999): Immunomodulatory activity of Unani gold preparations used in Indian systems of medicine. *Immunopharmacol. Immunotoxicol* **21(1)**, 151-62.

24. BAJAJ S, VOHORA SB (1998): Analgesic activity of gold preparations used in Ayurveda and Unani-Tibb. *Indian J., Med. Res.,* **108**, 104-11.

25. BAJAJ S, VOHORA SB (1999): Nootropic effects of Korean ginseng tea and calcined gold preparations used in Ayurveda and Unani-Tibb. *Internat Colloquium on Brain Research*, Indian National Science Academy, New Delhi.

26. BAJAJ S, VOHORA SB (1999): Anticataleptic, antianxiety and antidepressant activity of gold preparations used in Indian systems of medicine. *Internat Congress Frontiers Pharmacol Therap 21st Century*, New Delhi.

27. BALDUINI C, PECCI A, LOFFREDO G, IZZO P, NORIS P, GROSSO M, BERG MASCHI G, ROSTI V, MAGRINI U, CERESA IF, CONJI V, POGGI V, SOVOIA A (2004): Effects of R216Q mutation of GATA-1 on erythrocytosis and megakeratopoisis. *Thromb Haemost Pediatr.*, **91(1)**, 129-40.

28. BARLETT H, EPERJESTI F (2004): An ideal ocular nutritional supplement? *Ophthalmic Physiol Opt*, **24(4)**, 339-49.

29. BEHNE D (1991): Metabolism and biological functions of selenium. In: *Trace-89: Trace Elements in Health and Disease* (Eds.: Yuregir GT, Donma O, Kayrin L), pp. 1-10, Cukurova University, Adana.

30. BENDERDOUR M, HESS K, NZIETCHUENG MP, NABET P, BELLEVILLE F, DOUSSET B (1999): Boron and extracellular matrix. In: *New Aspects of Trace Element Research* (Eds : Abdulla M, Bost M, Gamon S, Arnaud S, Chazot G), pp.17-21, Smith-Gordon, London/Nishimura, Tokyo.

31. BHATNAGAR S, NATCHU UC (2004): Zinc in child health and disease. *Indian J. Pediatr.*, **71(11)**, 991-95.

32. BHATNAGAR S, BAHL R, SHARMA PK, KUMAR GT, SAXENA SK, BHAN MK (2004): Zinc with oral rehydration therapy reduces stool output and duration of diarrhea in hospitalized children: a randomized controlled trial. *Curr. Gastroenterol Rep.*, **38(1)**, 34-40.

33. BISSE E, EPTING T, BEIL A, LINDNGER G, LANG H, WIELAND H (2005): Reference values for serum silicon in adults. *Ann. Biochem.*, **337(1)**, 130-35.

34. BLONIARZ J, ZAREBA S, RAHNAMA M (2004): Examination of nickel and chromium contents in selected herbs, herbal fruit teas and their infusions. *Prz. egl. Lek.* (Polish), **61 Suppl. 3**, 58-62.

35. BOWEN HJM (1984): *Environmental Chemistry of Elements*, Academic Press, London.

36. BROZEK J (1965): *Human Body Composition: Approaches and Applications*, Symposia of the Society of Human Biology, Vol. 7, Pergamon Press, London.

37. BRUNO B, ROTTA M, GIACCONEL, MASSAIA M, BERTOLA A, BOCCADORO M (2004): New drug treatment for multiple myeloma. *Lancet*, **5(7)**, 430-42.

38. CARDELLI NF (1986): *Tin as a Vital Nutrient: Implications in Cancer Prophylaxis and other Physiological Processes*, CRC Press, Florida.

39. CHAFFMAN M, BROGDEN RN, HEEL RG, SPEIGHT TM, AVERY GS (1984): Auranofin : a preliminary review of its pharmacological properties and therapeutic use in rheumatoid arthritis. *Drugs* **27**, 327.

40. CHANDRA SV (1983): Psychiatric illness due to manganese poisoning. *Acta. Psychiatr. Scand.* **24(5)**, **Suppl. 1**, 417-20.

41. CHANG GK (1999): Dietary intake of essential micronutrients in China. In: *New Aspects of Trace Element Research* (Eds.: Abdulla M, Bost M, Gamon S, Arnaud P, Chazot G), pp. 28-32, Smith-Gordon, London/Nishimura, Tokyo.

42. CHANG LW (1996): *Toxicology of Metals*, CRC Press Inc/Lewis Publishers, Boca Raton, USA.

43. COMBS GF (2005): Current evidence and research needs to support a health claim for selenium and cancer prevention. *J. Nutr.*, **135(2)**, 347-47.

44. COON JJ, ERNST E (2004): Complementary and alternative therapies in the treatment of chronic hepatitis C: a systematic review. *J. Hepatol.*, **40(3)**, 491-500.

45. COUGHLIN JR, NIELSEN FH (1999): Advances in boron essentiality research: Symposium summary. In: *New Aspects of Trace Element Research* (Eds.: Abdulla M, Bost M, Gamon S, Arnaud P, Chazot G), pp. 33-41, Smith-Gordon, London/Nishimura, Tokyo.

46. DARZYNKIEWICZ K, GRACZYK A, OLESZKIEWICZ J, RADOMSKA K, SOKOLOWSKA M, SWIATKOWSKA E, WATRAS J (1995): Magnesium deficiency in Polish children and psychosomatic disturbances : Medical and psychological aspects. In: *Trace and Toxic Elements in Nutrition and Health* (Eds.: Abdulla M, Vohora SB, Athar M), pp. 325-29, Jamia Hamdard and Wiley Eastern Ltd., New Delhi.

47. DE BOECK M, KIRSCH-VOLDERS M, LISON D (2003): Cobalt and antimony genotoxicity and carcinogenicity. *Mutat. Res.*, **548(1-2)**, 127-28.

48. DESOIZE B (2004): Metals and metal compounds in cancer treatment. *Anticancer Res.*, **24(3a)**, 1529-44.

49. DIXIT RC, VERMA SR, NITNAWARE V, THACKER NP (2003): Heavy metal contamination in surface and ground water supply of an urban city. *Indian J. Environ. Hlth.*, **45(2)**, 107-12.

50. DOCK L, VAHTER M (1999): Metal toxicology. In: *General and Applied Toxicology* (Eds.: Ballanlyne B, Marrs T, Syversen T), Edn. 2, Vol. 3, pp. 2049-78, McMillan Reference Ltd., London.

51. DONLY KT, BROWN DJ (2005): Identify, protect and restore: emerging issues in approaching child's oral health. *Gen. Dent.*, **53(2)**, 106-10.

52. DUPONT CO (1999): Silicon and the treatment of child myopia. In: *New Aspects of Trace Element Research* (Eds.: Abdulla M, Bost M, Gamon S, Arnaud P, Chazot G), pp. 245-247, Smith-Gordon, London/Nishimura, Tokyo.

53. EBY GA (2005): Treatment of acute lymphatic leukemia using zinc adjuvant with chemotherapy and radiation: a case history and hypothesis. *Med. Hypotheses*, **64(6)**, 1124-26.

54. ERDAL S, BUCHANAN SN (2005): A quantitative look at fluorosis: fluoride exposure and intake in children using a health risk assessment approach. *Environ. Health Persp.*, **13(1)**, 111-17.

55. FAWZI W (2003): Micronutrients and human immunodeficiency virus type 1 disease progression among adults and children. *Clin. Infect. Dis.*, **33(Supp)**, S112-16.

56. FERNANDES JS, NUNO L, RIBEIRO H, LINDER J, PAREIRA D, CARVALHO E, RABACAL C, APONSO JS, PAREIRA JN, HALPERN MJ (1995): Magnesium in cardiology: Ischemic disease, arrhythmias and miteral valve prolapse. In: *Trace and Toxic Elements in Nutrition and Health.* (Eds.: Abdulla M, Vohora SB, Athar MA), pp. 402-404, Jamia Hamdard and Wiley Eastern Ltd., New Delhi.

57. FERNANDES JS, RIBEIRO H, NUNO L, PAREIRA D, LINDER J, RABACAL C, CARVALHO E, AFONSO JS, PAREIRA JN, HALPERN MJ (1995): Magnesium therapy in acute myocardial infarction. In: *Trace and Toxic Elements in Nutrition and Health.* (Eds.: Abdulla M, Vohora SB, Athar MA), pp 405-407, Jamia Hamdard and Wiley Eastern Ltd., New Delhi.

58. FRAUSTO DASILVA JJR, WILLIAMS RJP (1991): *The Biological Chemistry of Elements*, Clarendon Press, Oxford.

59. FRIEDEN E (1984): *Biochemistry of Essential Ultra-Trace Elements*, Plenum Press, New York.

60. FREELAND-GRAVES JH (1999): Manganese: development of dietary recommendations for an essential yet toxic trace element. In: *New Aspects of Trace Element Research* (Eds.: Abdulla M, Bost M, Gamon S, Arnaud P, Chazot G), pp. 22-27, Smith-Gorden, London/ Nishimura, Tokyo.

61. FURST DE (1983): Mechanism of action, pharmacology, clinical efficacy and side effects of auranofin: an orally administered organic gold compound for the treatment of rheumatoid arthritis. *Pharmacology* **3(5)**, 284-94.

62. GAMBLING L, Mc ARDLE HJ (2004): Iron, copper and fetal development. Proc. *Nutr. Soc.*, **63(4)**, 553-62.

63. GANOTRA KB (1992): Central nervous system effects of *Kushta Hartal Warqi*: an arsenic preparation used in Unani medicine, *M. Pharm. Thesis (Pharmacology)*, Jamia Hamdard, New Delhi.

64. GANOTRA KB, VOHORA SB (1993): Neuropsychopharmacological studies on Kushta Hartal: an arsenic preparation used in Unani medicine. *Internat J. Toxicol., Occupat. Environ., Hlth.*, **2(1)**, p.211, 124.

65. GAWTHORNE JM, HOWELL JM, WHITE CL (1981): *Trace Element Metabolism in Man and Animals (TEMA-4)*, Springer Verlag, Berlin.

66. GENETS S, KALE RK, BAQUER NZ (1999): Effect of vanadate, insulin and fenugreek (*Trigonella foenum graecum*) on creatine kinase levels in tissues of diabetic rats. *Indian J. Exp. Biol.*, **37**, 200-202.

67. GENET S, KALE RK, BAQUER NZ (2002): Alterations in anti-diabetic enzymes and oxidative damage in experimental diabetic rat tissues: effects of vanadate and fenugreek (*Trigonella foenum graecum*), *Mol. Cell. Biochem.*, **236**, 7-12.

68. GILLETTE-GUYONET S, ANDRIEU S, NOURHASHMEI F, DE LA GUERONNIERE V, GRADNIJEAN H, VELLAS B (2005): Cognitive impairment and composition of drinking water in women: findings of the EPIDOS study. *Amer. J. Clin. Nutr.*, **81(4)**, 897-902.

69. GLEESON M, NIEMAN DC, PEDERSEN BK (2004): Exercise, nutrition and immune function. *J.Sports Sci.*, **22(1)**, 115-25.

70. GOOD RA (1999): Zinc and immunities. In: *New Aspects of Trace Element Research* (Eds.: Abdulla M, Bost M, Gamon S, Arnaud P, Chazot G), pp. 277-280, Smith-Gordon, London/ Nishimura, Tokyo.

71. GOYER RA, KLAASSEN CD, WALKIES MP (1995): *Metal Toxicology*, Academic Press, New York.

72. GUERRERO-ROMERO F, RODRIGUEZ-MORAN M (2005): Complementary therapies for diabetes: the case for chromium, manganese and antioxidants. *Arch. Med. Res.*, **36(3)**, 250-57.

73. GUMINSKA M (1990): Environmental fluoride and human health: In: *New Horizons of Health Aspects of Elements* (Eds.: Vohora SB, Dobrowolski JW), pp. 57-77, Jamia Hamdard, New Delhi.

74. GUMUSLU S, ONER G (1995): Effect of cadmium on glucose-6-phosphate dehydrogenase activity in rat blood cells. In: *Trace and Toxic Elements in Nutrition and Health* (Eds.: Abdulla M, Vohora SB, Athar M), pp. 156-164, Jamia Hamdard and Wiley Eastern Ltd, New Delhi.

75. GUPTA BL, PRET A, BAQUER NZ (2004): Protective effects of sodium orthovanadate in diabetic reticulocytes and aging red blood cells of wistar rats. *J. Biosci.*, **29(1)**, 73-79.

76. GUPTA D, RAJU J, PRAKASH JR, BAQUER NZ (1999): Change in lipid profile, lipogenic and related enzymes in the livers of experimental diabetic rats: effects of insulin and vanadate. *Diabetes Res. Clin. Pract.*, **46**, 1-7.

77. GUPTA SK (2002): *Emergency Toxicology: Management of Common Poisons*, Narosa Publishing House, New Delhi.

78. HAMBIDGE KM (1974): The clinical significance of trace element deficiencies in man. *Proc. Nutr. Soc*. **31**, 249.

79. HAMDARD ME, VOHORA SB (1989): *Medical Elementology: Practical Applications*, Institute of History of Medicine and Medical Research, New Delhi.

80. HAMEED A, VOHORA SB (1987): Elementology of neuropsychiatric disorders. In: *Elements in Health and Disease* (Eds.: Said M, Rahman MA, D'Silva LA), pp. 615-23, Hamdard Foundation, Karachi.

81. HAMEED A, VOHORA SB (2001): *Skin Diseases: a Herbomineral Approach*, CBS Publishers Distributers, Delhi.

82. HASHIMOTO K, WHITEHURST CE, MATSUBAR AK, LIPSKEY E (1992): Immunomodulatory effects of therapeutic gold compounds. *J. Amer. Clin. Invest.*, **89**, 1839-48.

83. HAVARINASAB S, HAGGQUIST B, BJORN E, POLLARD KM, HULTMAN P (2005): Immuno-suppressive and autoimmune effects of themerosal in mice. *Toxicol. Appl. Pharmacol.*, **204(2)**, 109-21.

84. HIEN TV, HUONG NB, HUONG PM, DUC NB (2002): Radioprotective effects of vitexina for breast cancer patients undergoing radiotherapy with Cobalt-60. *Integr. Cancer Ther.*, **1(1)**, 38-44.

85. HORN N, TONNESEN T, HEYDORN K, DAMSGAARD E, KAITILA I (1995): The distribution of tissue copper and other trace elements in occipital horn syndrome. In: *Trace and Toxic Elements in Nutrition and Health* (Eds.: Abdulla M, Vohora SB, Athar M) pp. 53-59, Jamia Hamdard and Wiley Eastern Ltd, New Delhi.

86. HUANG JH, YANG CC, DING SJ, YENG M, KAO CT, CHOU MY (2005): Inflammatory cytokines reaction elicited by root-end filling materials. *J. Biomed Res. B: Appl. Biometer.*, **73(1)**, 123-28.

87. HUSSEIN MA (2003): Trials of arsenic trioxide in multiple myeloma. *Cancer Control*, **10(5)**, 370-74.

88. IMURA N, NAGANUMA A, SATCH M, CHEN JT (1988): Trace elements as useful tools for cancer chemotherapy In: *Essential and Toxic Trace Elements in Health and Disease* (Ed.: Prasad AS), pp. 443-456, Alan R Liss Inc, New York.

89. INSEL PA (1996): Analgesic-antipyretic and anti-inflammatory agents and drugs in the treatment of gout. In: *Goodman and Gilman's The Pharmacological Basis of Therapeutics*, (Eds: Hardman JG, Limbred LE, Malinoff PB, Ruddon RW, Gilman AG), pp. 644-646 Ed. 9, McGraw Hill, New York.

90. IRMAK MB, INCE G, OZTURK M, CETINAJALAY R (2003): Acquired tolerance of hepatocellular carcinoma cells to selenium deficiency: a selective survival mechanism? *Cancer Res.*, **63(20)**, 6707-15.

91. IYENGAR GV (1981): Human health and trace elements research: problems and prospects. Editorial. *The Science of Total Environment* **19**, 105.

92. IYENGAR GV (1982): *Elemental Composition of Human and Animal Milk*, IAEA/TEC. DOC 269, International Atomic Energy Agency, Vienna.

93. IYENGAR GV, KOLLMER WE, BOWEN HJM (1978): *The Elemental Composition of Human Tissues and Body Fluids*, Verlag Chemie, Weinheim.

94. JAKUPEC MA, KEPPLER BK (2004), Gallium and other main group metal compounds as antitumour agents. *Met. Ions. Biol. Sys.*, **42**, 425-62.

95. KABATA-PENDIAS A, PENDIAS H (1984): *Trace Elements in Soils and Plants*, p. 313 CRC Press Inc., Boca Raton, Florida.

96. KANOJIA RK (1998): Chromium induced reproductive impairment in female rats. *Ph.D Thesis (Toxicology)* Jamia Hamdard, New Delhi.

97. KIEFFER F (1989): The evidence of selenium essentiality in man. In: *Nutrition in Clinical Practice: Proceedings of 10th Congress ESPEN, Leipzig 1988* (Eds.: Hartig et al.), pp. 262-72, Karger, Basel, Switzerland.

98. KILIC E, SARAYMEN R, DOMIROGLU A, OK E (2004): Chromium and manganese levels in the scalp hair of normal and patients with breast cancer. *Biol. Trace Elem. Res.*, **102(1-2)**, 19-25.

99. KIM HS, LEE SS, HWANGO Y, AHN KD, LEE BK (2003): Cross sectional study of blood lead effects on iron status in Korean lead workers. *Nutrition*, **19(7-8)**, 571-76.

100. KIM HS, LEE SS, LEE GS, HWANGO Y, AHN KD, LEE BK (2004): The protective effect of delta-aminolevulinic acid dehydratase 1-2 and 2-2 isozymes against blood lead with higher hematologic parameters. *Environ. Hlth. Perspect*, **112(5)**, 538-41.

101. KINGMAN A, ALBER JW, AREZZO JC, GARABRANT DH, MICHALEK JE (2005): Amalgam exposure and neurological function. *Neurotoxicology*, **26(2),** 241-55.

102. KINYUA AM, KOFI-TSEKPO WM, TOLO F, KAMAU GN, JAMBA IO, EL-BUSAIDY HS (1999): Essential trace element analysis of traditional medicines used in anti-convulsant therapy. In: *New Aspects of Trace Element Research* (Eds.: Abdulla M, Bost, M, Gamon S, Arnaud P, Chazol-G), pp. 235-240, Smith-Gordon, London/Nishimura, Tokyo.

103. KRISHNAN SS, McLACHLAN DR, DALTON AJ, KRISHNAN B, PENTON SSA, HARRISON JE, KRUCK T (1988): *Essential and Toxic Elements in Human Health and Disease* (Ed.: Prasad S), pp. 645-59, Allan R Liss Inc, New York.

104. LEWIS AJ, WALTZ DT (1982): Immunopharmacology of gold. In: *Progress in Medicinal Chemistry* (Eds.: Ellis GP, West GB), vol. 19, pp. 1-59, Elsevier Biomedical Press, New York.

105. LIM Y, LEVY M, BRAY TM (2004): Dietary zinc alters early inflammatory responses during cutaneous wound healing in weanling CD-1 mice. *J. Nutr.*, **134(4)**, 811-16.

106. LIST A, BERAN M, DE PERSIA J, SLACK J, VEY N, ROSENFELD CS, GREENBERG P (2003): Opportunities for Trisenox (arsenic trioxide) in the treatment of myeloblastic hydromas. *Leukemia*, **17(8)**, 1499-1507.

107. LIU H, PROBST A, LIAO B (2005). Metal contamination of soils and crops affected by the Chenzou lead/zinc mine spill (Hunan, China). *Sci. Total Environ.*, **339(1-3)**, 153-66.

108. LOEPER J, FRAGNEY M (1978): The physiological role of silicon and its anti-atheromatons action. In: *Biochemistry of Silicon and Related Problems* (Eds.: Bendz G, Lindaquist I), pp. 281-306, Plenum Press, New York.

109. LOUWE RJ, McDERMOTT LN, SONKE JJ, TIELENBERG R, WENDLING M, VAN HERK MB, MIJNHEE BJ (2004): The long-term stability of silicon flat panel imaging devices for dosimetry purposes. *Med. Phys.*, **31(11)**, 2989-95.

110. LUKASKI HC (2004): Vitamin and mineral status: effects on physical performance. *Nutrition*, **20(7-8)**, 632-44.

111. MAHAWAR RS, JAIN S, VERMA NK, CHAKRABARTI SP (1991): Release of toxic metals into the environment from natural and man-made sources in India. In: *New Aspects of Trace Element Research* (Eds.: Abdulla M, Bost M, Gamon S, Arnaud P, Chazot G), pp. 159-62, Smith-Gordon, London/Nishimura, Tokyo.

112. MARTHALER JM (2003): Success and drawbacks in the caries preventive use of fluorides: lessons to be learnt from history. *Oral Hlth. Prev. Dent.*, **1(2)**, 129-40.

113. MASIRONI R (1975): Trace elements in water and health. *WRC Drinking Water Quality and Public Health*, WHO Geneva.

114. MATHUR N, BHATNAGAR P, NAGAR P, BIJARNIA MK (2005): Mutagenicity assessment of effluents from textile/dye industries of Sanganer, Jaipur (India): a case study. *Ecotoxicol. Environ. Sof.*, **61(1)**, 105-13.

115. McCARTY MF (2005): Neutraceutical resources for diabetes prevention: an update. *Med Hypotheses*, **64(1)**, 151-58.

116. McCARTY MF (2005): Chromium picolinate may favourably influence the vascular risk associated with smoking by combined costisol-induced insulin resistance. *Med. Hypotheses*, **64(6)**, 1220-24.

117. MENZES G, D'SOUZA HS, VENKATESH T (2003): Chronic lead poisoning in an adult battery worker. *Occupat. Med.* (London), **53(7)**, 476-78.

118. MERIAN E (1991): *Metals and Their Compounds in the Environment*, VCH, Weinheim.

119. MEYER CH, SEKUNDO W (2005): Nutritional supplementation to prevent cataract formation. *Dev. Ophthalmol.*, **38**, 103-19.

120. MERTZ W (1974): The newer essential trace elements: Chromium, Nickel, Vanadium and Silicon. *Proc. Nutr. Soc.*, **33(3)**, 307.

121. MILLER AC, BROOKS K, SMITH J, PAGE N (2004): Effect of military-relevent heavy metals: depleted uranium and heavy metal tungsten alloy on gene expression in human liver carcinoma cells. *Mol. Cell. Biochem.*, **255(1-2)**, 249-56.

122. MISHRA GV, VOHORA SB, ATHAR M (1995): Mercury and lead preparations used in Unani-Tibb (Greco-Arab Medicine): Are these safe? *J. Trace Elements Exptl. Med.*, **8(2)**, 145.

123. MISHRA GV, VOHORA SB, ATHAR M (1995): Mercury and lead preparations used in Unani-Tibb (Greco-Arab Medicine) Part II: Effects on behaviour, oxidative stress, and chromosomal aberrations. *Indian J. Toxicol.*, **2(1&2)**, 51.

124. MOHAMMAD S, TAHA A, BAMEZAI RNK, BASIR SF, BAQUER NZ (2004): Lower doses of vanadate in combination with *Trigonella* restore altered carbohydrate metabolism and anti-oxidant status in alloxan-diabetic rats. *Clinica Chimmica Acta*, **342**, 105-14.

125. MOHANRAJ R, AZEEZ PA, PRISCILLA T (2004): Heavy metals in airborne particulate matter of urban Coimbatore. *Arch. Environ. Contamin.*, **47(2)**, 162-67.

126. NADKARNI KM (1976): *The Indian Materia Medica*, Part II, pp 1-133, Popular Prakashan Pvt Ltd., Bombay.

127. NESBITT J (2004): Gamma knife radiosurgery: a patient-friendly procedure. *Axone*, **25(3)**, 23-27.

128. NESBIT MA, BOWL MR, HARDING B, ALI A, AYALA A, CROWE C, DOBBIE A, HAMPSON G, HOLDAWAY I, LEVINE MA, McWILLIAMS R, SAMPSON J, WILLIAMS AJ, THAKKER RV (2004): Characterization of GATA 3 mutations in the hypoparathysoidism, deafness and renal dysplasia (HDR) syndrome. *J. Biol. Chem.*, **279(21)**, 22624-634.

129. NEUMANN CG, BWIBO NO, MURPHY SP, SIGMAN M, WHALEY S, ALLEN LH, GUTHRIE D, WEISS RE, DEMMENT MW (2003): Animal source foods improve dietary quality, micronutrient status, growth and cognitive function in Kenyan school children: background, study design and baseline findings. *J. Nutr.*, **133(11 Suppl. 2)**, 39413-495.

130. NEWNHAM RE (1984): *TEMA-5 Symposium on Trace Elements in Man and Animals*, pp. 839-841, Aberdeen.

131. NEWNHAM RE (1987): *Arthritis and Rheumatism Natural Health Association*, New Zealand. Personal communication.

132. NIELSEN FH (1980): Personal communication.

133. NIELSEN FH (1988): The ultra-trace elements. In: *Trace Minerals in Foods* (Ed. Smith KT), pp. 357-423, Marcel Dekker, New York.

134. NIELSEN FH (1996): The evidence for the nutritional essentiality of boron. *J. Trace .Elem., Exp. Med.* **9**, 215-29.

135. NIELSEN FH, PENLAND JG (1995): Clinical and biological consequences of boron deprivation in humans. In: *Trace and Toxic Elements in Nutrition and Health* (Eds.: Abdulla M, Vohora SB, Athar M), pp. 361-74, Jamia Hamdard and Wiley Eastern Ltd., New Delhi.

136. OH R (2005): Practical applications of fish oil (Omega-3 fatty acids) in primary care. *J. Amer. Board Fam. Pract.*, **18(1)**, 28-36.

137. OHYE C, SHIBAZAKI T, SATO S (2005): Gamma knife thalamotomy for movement disorders: evaluation of thalamic lesion and clinical results. *J. Neurosurg*, **102(Suppl.)**, 234-50.

138. ONER G, SENTURK UK (1995): Role of cholesterol in manganese-induced learning defects. In: *Trace and Toxic Elements in Nutrition and Health* (Eds.: Abdulla M, Vohora SB, Athar M), pp 147-151, Jamia Hamdard and Wiley Eastern Ltd., New Delhi.

139. ONO T, WADA O, YAMAMOTO M (1992): Study on the essentiality of lithium. *Biomed. Res. Trace Elem.*, **3**, 41-47.

140. PARR RM, IYENGAR GV (1999): The role of minerals and trace elements in osteoporosis. In: *New Aspects of Trace Element Research* (Eds.: Abdulla M, Bost M, Gamon S, Arnaud P, Chazot G), pp. 148-152, Smith-Gordon, London/Nishimura, Tokyo.

141. PATEL AB, DHANDE LA, RAWAT MS (2003): Economic evaluation of zinc and copper use in treating acute diarrohea in children: a randomized controlled trial. *Cost Eff. Resour. Alloc.*, **1(1)**, 7-9.

142. PERRY HM (1971): Trace elements related to cardiovascular disease. In: *Environmental Geochemistry in Health and Disease* (Eds.: Cannon HL, Hopps HC), pp. 179-96, The Geological Society of America, Colorado.

143. PETERSEN PE, LENNON MA (2004): Effective use of fluorides for the prevention of dental caries in the 21st century: the WHO approach. *Community Dent. Oral Epidemiol.*, **32(5)**, 319-21.

144. PICHARDO D, SINGHAL S, MEHTA J, ROSEN S (2003): Recent developments and future directions in the treatment of multiple myeloma. *Cancer Biother. Radiopharm.*, **18(4)**, 497-511.

145. PRASAD AS (1988): *Essential and Toxic Elements in Human Health and Disease*, Alan R Liss Inc, New York.

146. RAHMAN MJ, SARKAR P, ROY SK, AHMAD SM, CHISTI J, AZIM T, MATHAN M, SACK D, ANDERSSON J, RAQIB R (2005): Effects of zinc supplementation as adjuvant therapy on the systemic immune responses in shigellosis. *Amer. J. Clin. Nutr.*, **81(2)**, 495-502.

147. RAI V, AGNIHOTRI AK, KHATOON S, RAWAT AK, MEHROTRA S (2005): Chromium in some herbal drugs. *Bull. Environ. Contamin. Toxicol.*, **74(3)**, 464-69.

148. RAJPATHAK S, RIMM EB, LI T, MORRIS JS, STAMPFER MJ, WILLEJ WC, HU FB (2004): Lower toenail chromium in men with diabetes and cardiovascular disease compared with healthy men. *Diabetes Care*, **27(9)**, 2211-16.

149. REDOL GS, REIS MF (1995): The role of copper ions in infection and inflammation. In: *Trace and Toxic Elements in Nutrition and Health* (Eds.: Abdulla M, Vohora SB, Athar M), pp 107-11, Jamia Hamdard and Wiley Eastern Ltd., New Delhi.

150. RIBEIRO DA, MARQIES ME, DE ASSIS GF, ANZAI A, POLETI ML, SALVADORI DM (2004): No relationship between subchronic fluoride intake and DNA damage in Wistar rats. *Caries Res.*, **38(6)**, 576-79.

151. RIZVI SNA, RIZVI SSA (1987): Comparative clinical evaluation of a new Unani oral hypoglycemic agent *Kushta Hartal* (*Tabqi*) and chlorpropamide in maturity onset diabetes mellitus. *First International Seminar on Unani Medicine*, Abstract p. 30, WHO and Central Council for Research in Unani Medicine, New Delhi.

152. ROY RK, KAPOOR DN, NATH SS (1974): Marginal leakage of silver amalgam restorations. *J. Indian Dentl. Ass.*, **46(5)**, 195-99.

153. SAGLAM AM, BAYSAL V, CEYLAN AM (2004): Nickel and cobalt hypersensitivity reaction before and after orthodontic therapy in children. *J. Contemp. Dent. Pract.*, **5(4)**, 79-90.

154. SAID M (1969): *Hamdard Pharmacopoeia of Eastern Medicine*, pp. 222-34, Hamdard Foundation, Karachi.

155. SAID M, RAHMAN MA, ABDULLA M, VOHORA SB, ATHAR M (1996). *Elements and Liver*, Hamdard Foundation, Karachi.

156. SATARUG S, MOORE MR (2004): Adverse health effects of chronic low-level cadmium in foodstuffs and cigarette smoke. *Environ. Hlth. Perspect*, **112(10)**, 1099-1103.

157. SAUNDERS LZ (1983): The toxicology of auranofin. *International Symposium on Auranofin*, Excerpta Medica, Amsterdam.

158. SCHROEDER HA (1976): *The Trace Elements and Nutrition: Some Positive and Negative Aspects*, Faber and Faber, London.

159. SENTURK UK, ONER G, IZGUT VN (1995): The mechanism of cadmium-induced hypertension in rats. In: *Trace and Toxic Elements in Nutrition and Health* (Eds.: Abdulla M, Vohora SB, Athar M), pp. 152-55, Jamia Hamdard and Wiley Eastern Ltd., New Delhi.

160. SHAH NF (1985): *Kushta-e-Jat: Tarkib wa Istemal* (Urdu), p. 113, Muktaba al Jaisat, Rampur.

161. SHAH SA, VOHORA SB (1990): Boron enhances anti-arthritic effects of garlic oil. *Fitoterapia* **56(2)**, 121-26.

162. SHAH ZA (2001): Investigations on some plant and mineral origin drugs for protective action against stress and ischemic brain injury. *Ph.D. Thesis (Toxicology)*, Jamia Hamdard, New Delhi.

163. SHAH ZA, VOHORA SB (2002): Antioxidant/restorative effects of calcined gold preparations used in Indian systems of medicine against global and focal models of ischemia. *Pharmacol. & Toxicol.*, **90**, 254-59.

164. SHAH ZA, SHARMA P, VOHORA SB (2005): Attenuation of stress-elicited brain catecholamines, serotonin and plasma conticosterone levels by calcined gold preparations used in Indian systems of medicine. *Pharmacol. & Toxicol.*, **96**, 469-74.

165. SHEN ZX, CHEN CQ, NI JH, LI XS, XIONG SM, QIU OY, ZHU J, JANG W, SUN GL, YANG KQ, CHEN Y, ZHOU L, FANG ZW, WANG YT, MA J, ZHANG P, ZHANG TD,

CHEN SJ, CHEN Z, WANG ZY (1997): Use of arsenic tri-oxide (As_2O_3) in the treatment of acute granulocytic leukemia (APL). II Clinical efficacy and pharmacokinetics in relapsed patients. *Blood* **89**, 3354-60.

166. SHEN ZX, SHI ZZ, FANG J, GU BW LI YM, SHI JY, ZHENG PZ, YAN H, LIU YF, CHEN Y, SHEN Y, WU W, TANJ W, WAXMAN S, DE THE H, WANG ZY, CHEN SJ, CHEN Z (2004): All-transretionoic acid/As_2 O_3 combination yields a high quality remission and survival in newly diagnosed acute promyelocytic leukemia. *Proc. Natl. Acad. Sci. USA*, **101(15)**, 5328-35.

167. SIDDIQUI R (2000). Neuropsychopharmacological and Immunomodulating studies on calcined arsenic and lead preparations used in Unani-Tibb. *Ph.D. Thesis (Toxicology)*, Jamia Hamdard, New Delhi.

168. SIDDIQUI R, VOHORA SB (1999): Neuropsychopharmacological profile of *Kushta-e-Musallus*, calcined lead preparation used in Greco-Arab system of medicine. *Internat. Colloquium on Brain Research*, Indian National Science Academy, New Delhi.

169. SIDDIQUI R, VOHORA D, VOHORA SB (1999): Proconvulsant effects of calcined arsenic preparations used in Indian systems of medicine. *Indian J. Pharmacol.*, **31**, 150-2.

170. SIDDIQUI R, MISHRA GV, VOHORA SB (2002): Effect of therapeutic doses of calcined arsenic and lead preparations in rats. *Indian J. Vet. Pathol.*, **26(1,2)**, 81-82.

171. SIDDIQUI R, VOHORA SB (2004): Studies on calcined arsenic preparations used in Indian systems of medicine for effects on anxiety and depression. *Toxicol. Internat.*, **11(1)**, 43-47.

172. SINGH NP, WRENN ME (1999): The metabolic and pathological aspects of uranium. In: *Metabolism of Minerals and Trace Elements in Human Disease* (Eds.: Abdulla M, Dashti H, Sarkar B, Al-Sayer H, Al-Naqeeb N), pp. 163-69, Smith-Gordon, London/Nishimura, Tokyo.

173. SMALL EJ, HALABI S, DALBAGNI G, PURUTHI R, PHILLIPS G, EDELMAN M, BAJORIN D (2003): Overview of bladder cancer trials in the cancer and leukemia group B. *Cancer*, **97(8 Suppl.)**, 2090-98.

174. SMITH HA (1984): Cadmium. In: *Biochemistry of the Essential Ultra-Trace Elements* (Ed.: Frieden E), p. 361, Plenum Press, New York.

175. SMITH KM, SAHYOUN NR (2005): Fish consumption: recommendations versus advisories, can they be reconciled? *Nutr. Rev.*, **63(2)**, 39-46.

176. SOWDEN E, PIPIE A (1958): Barium and strontium concentrations in eye tissues. *Biochem. J.*, **70**, 716-720.

177. SRIVASTAVA AK, GUPTA BN (1996): Role of selenium in health and disease. *Indian J. Clin. Pract.*, **6(8)**, 32-39.

178. SRIVASTAVA P, SAXENA AK, KALE RK, BAQUER NZ (1995): Antidiabetogenic role of lithium. In: *Trace and Toxic Elements in Nutrition and Health* (Eds.: Abdulla M, Vohora SB, Athar M), pp. 392-95, Jamia Hamdard and Wiley Eastern Ltd., New Delhi.

179. STAESSEN JA, ROELS HA, EMELIANOY D, KUZNETSOVA J, THIJS I, VANGRONSVELD J, FAGARD R (1999): Environmental exposure to cadmium, forearm density and risk of fractures: prospective population study, *Lancet* **353**, 1140-44.

180. SUSHEELA AK (1999): Fluorosis management programme in India: The impact of networking between health and rural drinking water supply implementing agencies, In: *Toxicology and Environmental Health* (Eds.: Vohora SB and Agarwal VP), pp. 125-36, Society for Biosciences and Jamia Hamdard, New Delhi.

181. SZYMANSKA-CHABOWSKA A, ANTONWICZ-JUCHNIEWICZ J, ANDRZEJAK R (2004): Plasma concentration of selected neoplastic markers in persons occupationally exposed to arsenic and heavy metal. *Med. Pract.*, **55(4)**, 313-20.

182. TALWAR GP (1980): *Textbook of Biochemistry & Biology*. Prentice-Hall of India Pvt Ltd.; New Delhi.

183. TANDI NK, NYAMANGARA J, BANGIRA C (2004): Environmental and potential health effects of growing leafy vegetables on soil irrigated using sewage sludge and effluent; a case of Zn and Cu. *J. Environ. Sci. Hlth.*, **39(3)**, 561-71.

184. TRAVACIO M, POLO JM, CONTE I, LLESUY S (1999): Oxidative stress-induced by Chromium (VI). *New Aspects of Trace Element Research* (Eds.: Abdulla M, Bost M, Gamon S, Arnaud P, Chazot G), pp 178-83, Smith-Gordon London/Nishimura, Tokyo.

185. TYRER SP, DELVES HJ, WELLER MP (1979): CSF copper in schizophrenia. *Amer. J. Psychiatry* **116(7)**, 917-21.

186. UMESH CS, YADAV K, MOORTHY, BAQUER NZ (2005): Combined treatment of sodium orthovanadate and *Momordica charantia* fruit extract prevents alterations in lipid profile and lipogenic enzymes in diabetic rats. *Mol. Cell Biochem.*, **268**, 111-20.

187. UNDERWOOD EJ (1971): *Trace Elements in Human and Animal Nutrition*, Academic Press, New York.

188. UNNIKRISHNAN D, LUCARIELLO R, WIERNIL PH (2004): Cardiac monitoring of patients receiving arsenic trioxide therapy. *Brit. J. Hematol.*, **124(5)**, 610-17.

189. USAL A, ACATURK E, TETIKER T, ARPACI A, YUREGER GT (1995): Serum magnesium and potassium levels in digitalized patients. In: *Trace and Toxic Elements in Nutrition and Health* (Eds : Abdulla M, Vohora SB, Athar M), pp. 413-18, Jamia Hamdard and Wiley Eastern Ltd., New Delhi.

190. VAHTER M (1988): *In vivo* methylation and detoxification of arsenic. In: *The Biological Alkylation of Metals* (Eds.: Craig PJ, Glockling F), The Royal Society of Chemistry, London.

191. VERMA A, KANWAR KC (1999): Trace elements in the seminal plasma of normospermic, oligospermic and azoospermic males. *Trace Elements & Electrolytes* **16(3)**, 135-36.

192. VOHORA D, VOHORA SB (1999): Elemental basis of epilepsy. *Trace Elements & Electrolytes*, Germany **16**, 109-23.

193. VOHORA SB (1982): Is human body a microcosm? In: *Earth, Elements and Man*, pp. 27-52, Institute of History of Medicine and Medical Research, New Delhi.

194. VOHORA SB (1982): Elements in human health and disease. In: *Earth, Elements and Man, Supplement-1*, pp. 1-18, Institute of History of Medicine and Medical Research, New Delhi.

195. VOHORA SB (1983): *Medical Elementology*, Institute of History of Medicine and Medical Research, New Delhi.

196. VOHORA SB (1984): Medical Elementology: birth of a new discipline in science. *Curare* Germany **7(3)**, 155.

197. VOHORA SB (1986): Elementology of leprosy. *Indian J. Lepr*. **58(3)**, 451.

198. VOHORA SB (1996): Elementology of liver diseases and alcoholism. In: *Elements and Liver* (Eds.: Said M, Rahman MA, Abdulla M, Vohora SB, Athar M), pp. 111-27, Hamdard Foundation, Karachi.

199. VOHORA SB, AGARWAL VP (1999): *Toxicology and Environmental Health*, Asiatech Publishers Inc., Delhi.

200. VOHORA SB, DOBROLWOLSKI JW (1990): *New Horizons of Health Aspects of Elements*, Jamia Hamdard, New Delhi.

201. VOHORA SB, KIM HS, SHAH SA, KHANNA T, DANDIYA PC (1991): CNS and adaptogenic effects of *Siddha Makardhwaja* an Ayurvedic mercury preparation. *Internat. J. Toxicol. Occupat. Environ. Hlth.*, **1(1)**, P1, 103.

202. VOHORA SB, SIDDIQUI R, VOHORA D (1999): Role of magnesium in neuropsychiatric disorders and cognitive functions. *Biol. Magnezol. Poland.*, **4**, 236-40.

203. WANG H (1999): Toxic effects of cadmium and selenium on the nutritional elements In: *New Aspects of Trace Element Research* (Eds.: Abdulla M, Bost M, Gamon S, Arnaud P, Chazot G), pp. 92-94, Smith-Gordon, London/ Nishimura, Tokyo.

204. WANG Z, ZHOU J, LU X, GONG Z, LE XC (2004): Arsenic speciation in urine from acute myelocytic leukemia patients undergoing arsenic trioxide treatment. *Chem. Res. Toxicol.*, **17(1)**, 95-103.

205. WAXMAN S, ANDERSON KC (2001): History of the development of arsenic derivatives in cancer therapy. *Oncologist*, **6(Suppl. 2)**, 3-10.

206. WELLIUM GR, ZAMENHOFF RG, TOPLIN EL (1982): Boron neutron capture radiation therapy of cerebral gliomas: an analysis of possible use of boron-induced antibodies for selective concentration of boron in gliomas. *Internat. J. Radiat. Oncol. Biol. Phys.*, **8(8)**, 1339-47.

207. WESTER PO (1989): Magnesium and cardiovascular disease. In: *Metabolism of Minerals and Trace Elements in Human Disease* (Eds.: Abdulla M, Dashti H, Sarkar B, Al-Sayer H, Al-Naqeeb N), pp. 1-10, Smith-Gordon, London/Nishimura, Tokyo.

208. WHO (1984): *Guidelines for Drinking Water Quality*, Vols.1 & 2, World Health Organization, Geneva.

209. WHO (1996): *Trace Elements in Human Nutrition and Health*, World Health Organization, Geneva.

210. WIDDOWSON EM (1965): Chemical analysis of human body. In: *Human Body Composition: Approaches and Applications* (Ed. Brozek J.), pp. 31-48, Pergamon Press, New York.

211. WIDDOWSON EM, DICKERSON JWJ (1964): Chemical composition of the body. In: *Mineral Metabolism: An Advanced Treatise* (Eds., Comor CL and Bronner F), Vol. 2, Part A, pp. 222-48, Academic Press, New York.

212. WILLIAMS DR (1971): *The Metals of Life*, pp. 4-5, Von Nostrand Reinhald Co., London.

213. WOOD JP, OSBORNE NN (2003): Zinc and energy requirements in induction of oxidative stress to retinal pigmented epithelial cells. *Neurochem. Res.*, **28(10)**, 1525-33.

214. XIONG ZT, WANG H (2005): Copper toxicity and bioaccumulation in Chinese cabbage (*Brassica pekinensis* Rupr), *Environ. Toxicol.*, **20(2)**, 188-94.

215. YOSHIDA C, MELO JV (2004): Biology of chronic myeloid leukemia and possible approaches to imatinib-resistant disease. *Int. J. Hematol.*, **79(5)**, 420-33.

216. YOSHIDA T, SHIMAMURA T, SHIGETA S (1987): Enhancement of immune response *in vitro* by arsenic. *Internat. J. Immunotoxicology,* **9**, 411-15.

217. YUREGIR GT, DONMA O, KAYRIN L (1991): *Trace'89: Proceedings of the Third International Congress on Trace Elements in Health and Disease*, Medical Faculty, Cukurova University, Adana, Turkey.

218. ZAICHICK V (1999): Human intrathyroid iodine in health and non-thyroid disease. In: *New Aspects of Trace Element Research* (Eds.: Abdulla M, Bost M, Gamon S, Arnaud P, Chacot G), pp 114-19, Smith-Gordon, London/Nishimura, Tokyo.

219. ZELIKOFF JT, COHEN MD (1996): Immunotoxicology of inorganic metal compounds. In: *Experimental Immunotoxicology* (Eds : Smialowicz RJ, Holsopple MP), pp. 189-228, CRC Press Inc., Boca Raton.

220. ZHUK LI, KIST AA, MUSABAEV EL, DZ HURAE V RKH, YASHINA TY, BARNOUN J, DANILOVA EA (1999): Selenium and other elements in viral hepatitis. In: *New Aspects of Trace Element Research* (Eds.: Abdulla M, Bost M, Gamon S, Arnaud P, Chazot G), pp. 261-65, Smith-Gordon, London/Nishimura, Tokyo.

AUTHOR

Shashi B. Vohora, M.V.Sc., Ph.D., D.Sc. retired as Professor and Head of the Department of Medical Elementology and Toxicology, Jamia Hamdard (Hamdard University), New Delhi. He was earlier working for the Indian Council of Medical Research, at the Post-graduate Institute of Medical Education and Research, Chandigarh, Lady Hardinge Medical College, New Delhi and later for the Institute of History of Medicine and Medical Research, New Delhi. He has over 30 years of Teaching/Research/Editing experience and about 200 research publications including 16 books. His papers have been cited in books published from USA and some publications were translated into Polish, Italian and Hungarian languages. He is the first Ph.D. in Science Policy in India. His major areas of interest are Neuro-psycho-behavioural studies, Medicinal Plants, Medical Elementology and Traditional Mineral Drugs. He was awarded research projects by the Indian Council of Medical Research, Central Council for Research in Unani Medicine University Grants Commission, and the Department of Science and Technology, Government of India on neuropsychopharmacological, immunomodulatory studies and on hypoperfusion/ reperfusion-induced brain injury. Two M. Pharm. (1991, 1992) and eight Ph.D. (1993 to 2002) degrees were awarded under his supervision. One candidate carried out post-doctoral research under his guidance with Research Associateship from the Council of Scientific and Industrial Research. Prof. Vohora has participated in many national and international conferences and was Organizing Secretary of the IHMMR/WHO sponsored First International Conference on Elements in Health and Disease, New Delhi (1983), National Symposium on the Development of Indigenous Drugs in India during the last 25 Years, New Delhi (1988), International Symposium on New Drug Development, New Delhi (1998), and Convener of the National Symposium on Toxicology and Environmental Health, New Delhi (1998). He has been on scientific visits/academic tours to Poland, Hungary, Germany, France, Switzerland, Italy, Sri Lanka, Pakistan and Nepal and has delivered several invited/plenary lectures in India and abroad. He is a nominated member of the Board of Governers, Ansted University, Virgin Islands, UK. Founder member and Promoter of the International Union of Elementologists and member of International Brain Research Organization, France, International Society for Trace Element Research in Humans, USA. Indian Pharmacological Society, Society of Biosciences India and Correspondent Member *Curare*, Germany and *Investigational Drugs*, UK.

Address : 114 Kailash Hills, New Delhi 110 065, India.
sbvohora31@rediffmail.com